THE NEXT TRILLION DOLLAR INDUSTRY

THE RETAIL HEALTHCARE REVOLUTION

HOW EMPOWERED HEALTHCARE
CONSUMERS ARE CREATING
THE WORLD'S LARGEST RETAIL MARKET

TONY PAQUIN

The Retail Healthcare Revolution
Tony Paquin

1. Title 2. Author 3. Healthcare

Library of Congress Control Number: 2009925257

ISBN 10: 0-9824239-0-X
ISBN 13: 978-0-9824239-0-5

For Anthony and Madison,
because all I do, I do for you

CONTENTS

ACKNOWLEDGEMENTS

Like many good business ideas, retail healthcare was born out of an "a-ha" moment. Several years ago, I was leading a consulting engagement with a very large not-for-profit health system in Florida. At that time, the hospital was evaluating how to best optimize hundreds of acres of land surrounding their large tertiary facility. The vision morphed into a focused retail village to address the health and lifestyle needs of the whole person. Healthy restaurants, fitness facilities, medical spas, vitamin shops, as well as physicians' offices would all be interspersed in a "shopping" district of sorts. Up to this point, this concept was unheard of in healthcare. It was a turning point for me. The further I investigated, it became apparent that there were numerous unmet retail needs of everyday patients and consumers; and clearly, hospital systems were in the best position to effectively meet those needs. Also, it was obvious that the healthcare industry would need to embrace new business models in light of coming financial pressures caused by the aging Baby Boomer generation. Financial success for healthcare systems in the early twenty-first century will require a consumer focus unheard of in the previous fifty years.

As a result, Paquin Healthcare Companies was formed in 2005 with the goal of coaching hospital executives across the country on best practices in retail healthcare solutions and positively impacting the financial viability of the healthcare industry.

This book simply would not have been possible without the support of some very special people who have supported my passion for retail healthcare and consistently encouraged my pursuit of documenting this story. Acknowledgments go to the entire team at Paquin Healthcare who support our company everyday. First and foremost, I have been fortunate to have Gary Paquin, my brother, best friend and business partner working alongside me to build the vision for serving our clients. Gary's background in business development and skill at building relationships has been a huge asset in expanding retail healthcare into the C-Suite of hospitals.

I would also like to recognize Gina Andrews, who was the first employee hired at Paquin Healthcare and currently serves as my Executive Assistant and Office Manager. Gina was instrumental in proofreading the book, keeping the project on task, and overseeing a number of rewrites of the manuscript. Gina's attention to detail, as well as, her strong support during this entire process is deeply valued.

My thanks go to Gloria Caulfield, our Vice President of Marketing, for her editing and ongoing feedback on the manuscript. Gloria is a proven healthcare professional with keen insights into healthcare marketing. Her support in managing the entire book publishing process — from writing to final printing has been invaluable.

Our Graphics Manager, Crystal Aria, is a talented and creative professional that has provided excellent branding and design work on numerous projects for our clients. Crystal is known in our office for going the extra mile and has done it again by exceeding my expectations on the book's typesetting and cover design. Crystal's commitment to this project has been stellar.

Over the years, Paquin Healthcare has been blessed with strong business relationships and valuable strategic partners. Several of our partners have contributed content and provided interviews to *The Retail Healthcare Revolution*. To each of our contributors, those that took time to share your wisdom, thank you for your thought leadership. Our story would simply not be as compelling without your support. Thanks for working with us everyday to deliver the best possible retail solutions to our healthcare clients.

Most importantly, I would like to say thank you to all of our clients; over 200 and growing! I deeply appreciate the friendships that we have formed during the journey, as well as the opportunity to work with so many well-respected medical institutions around the country. Thank you for supporting Paquin Healthcare and collaborating with us to pioneer a new retail channel. Together, we have had many successes and key discoveries. One thing I am very sure of is that we are only scratching the surface in retail healthcare and the best is yet to come.

THE BUSINESS OF HEALTHCARE: A TERMINAL PROGNOSIS

Imagine the United States' healthcare system as a patient visiting a doctor. Dragging itself into the office, the once-vital institution is plagued by an assortment of maladies, each symptom weakening it further, each treatment slowly but surely draining its energy and financial resources.

The doctor conducts a thorough exam, carefully gauging the patient's vital signs, and is ready to deliver his grim prognosis.

"You should have come to me for a solution sooner," he reports. "You have very little time left."

It's a metaphor, of course, but an entirely apt one. The longstanding healthcare system in the United States is in its death throes, a terminal patient whose well-being has been neglected for far too long, whether the majority of those dependent on it realize it or not. What's missing is a wholesale acknowledgement of the new dynamic by both the industry and the public, and a systemic, adaptive response to the changes taking place.

This patient, the U.S. healthcare system, can't be cured, but it can be taught to adapt. There is a solution, but it requires fast action and decisive thinking. In order for healthcare as an institution to continue to function in the United States in a manner that meets the needs of both the providers and the public, it *must* change, and it must change *now*. This is not a suggestion any more than a stroke is a mere suggestion that one should stop smoking. Time is of the essence.

Change is inevitable in any system, and seismic shifts in the American healthcare industry in recent years have included cuts to Medicare, the increasingly high cost of health insurance, the growing number of uninsured and underinsured Americans and the economic collapse of the traditional, reimbursement-based healthcare system. These are the obvious, negative changes — the shifts we're becoming cognizant of as the system becomes progressively more difficult to navigate for both patients and healthcare providers.

But there are also positive, less-obvious changes occurring in healthcare at a cultural level. For starters, Americans have never been better informed about their healthcare options and, in general, are more proactive in caring for themselves, eschewing smoking and saturated fats, getting more exercise and supplementing their diets as needed. Healthcare information, once accessible only to medical professionals, has moved into the public domain and many individuals access this knowledge to proactively maintain their health.

Educated and proactive Americans no longer see themselves as patients who only consult medical experts when they need critical care. They are consumers who are informed about the choices available to them; they make healthcare decisions based on their informed opinions and, increasingly, spend money on maintaining their wellness.

More and more, healthcare consumers don't automatically default to their doctors. They research their options, get second opinions and address their wellness in a proactive rather than reactive manner. To a healthcare consumer, doctors and hospitals are no longer last-resort options — they are resources for maintaining a healthy life.

As a result, the retail end of healthcare, the over-the-counter, cash-in-hand business of providing wellness, has exploded, just as the reimbursement-based system has seemingly exhausted its sustainability.

The medical establishment has been slow to recognize this shift from patient to consumer. Those institutions that recognize their patients as informed, discriminating consumers have transitioned to providing wellness options in addition to traditional acute care. This isn't merely an option for augmenting existing healthcare institutions; it's essential to survival.

Survival is important these days, too, when one-third of all American hospitals currently operate at a loss, making their long-term prognoses grim. Many hospitals are closing not for a lack of patients — there are a surplus of those — but because the current system is economically untenable. Another one-third of American hospitals essentially break even, which may keep them in business but still shows how vulnerable any medical institution can be to collapsing. The final third make a profit, but on average it is single-digit — hardly a harbinger of future success in an already dismal market. This financial pressure is caused by reduced reimbursement payments that hospitals receive for their services.

Reimbursement-based medicine has several drawbacks, none more apparent than the disproportionate number of people paying into the system. When considering the impending insolvency of Medicare, for example, one need look no further than the number of wage earners paying into the system: In 1950 there were sixteen people paying in for every individual collecting benefits; today that ratio is three-to-one, and by 2030 it will be an even two-to-one.

When traditional medicine was solvent there was no need to look for alternative ways to enhance earnings. Twenty years ago most physicians would have recoiled at the notion of integrating their existing practices with retail operations because the system worked for them as it was. However, today's reimbursement-based system is so thoroughly inefficient that retail has become an industry salvation for those who recognize its value.

Just as Wal-Mart brought healthcare into the retail industry, modern hospitals, clinics and medical practices are bringing retail into the healthcare business. Hospitals once relied almost exclusively on their patients' need for acute care, but that's no longer true. Patients are now also consumers who are hungry for information, services and products. Hospitals that decline to provide what consumers want will invariably lose business to more forward-thinking companies. In fact, most consumers seeking health-related products and services are more healthy than they are sick or injured, and as a result are looking for "health" solutions not "sick care" solutions.

The term "healthcare" has often been used inappropriately. Traditional medicine is actually "sick care"; that is, it treats illness rather than teaching and maintaining wellness. What we know as "healthcare" today has evolved as the industry has come to recognize the value of prevention and as consumers have sought ways to stay healthy rather than merely treating sicknesses and injuries

— the results of not addressing the care of their health, as was the tradition in the old healthcare industry model. Consumers are looking for healthcare solutions that are more relevant to today's economic and clinical environment.

Some of the purveyors in the exploding field of healthcare are less informed, less reliable and less convenient than consumers deserve and desire. Health and wellness has become a free-market economy, an economic Wild West with thousands of players and billions of dollars at stake. And only the institutions that adapt to economic realities will survive in this new paradigm.

One way to do that is to focus on retail success, which is built around providing people with attractive options. For example, Wal-Mart's offering of discounted generic prescriptions, which tests the conventional pharmacy model, and hospitals offering branded vitamins and healthcare products, which similarly tests the conventional retailer system. Unlike the reimbursement-based healthcare system, retail-based, wellness-oriented healthcare is economically sound, and it's growing at an astonishing pace.

The goal of retail healthcare is to provide more productive business practices for all healthcare providers and to create more and better healthcare options for consumers. More choices for consumers means healthier, happier customers, which in turn means more economic prosperity for those who can provide those choices. The definition of a good business arrangement is one in which all parties benefit, and healthcare providers who can fulfill their mission of serving both individuals and the community as a whole will find financial success.

This revolution in healthcare isn't some futuristic projection. It's happening now in healthcare facilities across the United States.

Now, let's look at how to put our metaphorical patient back on the road to wellness.

CHAPTER 1

CONSUMERS IN CONTROL

How has healthcare changed in recent years? The obvious examples are advances in pharmacology and technology. We marvel at innovations in surgery and consider the possibilities lying in the decoded human genome. Our elderly live longer, more fulfilling lives. Fifty, as they say, is the new forty.

But subtle changes have also occurred in how patients view their care. It wasn't long ago that many people could claim to have spent only one day in the hospital: the day they were born. For most twentieth-century consumers, doctors were the primary sources of care and hospitals the destinations of last resort. Patients were largely responsible for their own care — but only to the extent that they followed their doctors' instructions.

Looking back a little further, hospitals weren't even common until the nineteenth century. Prior to that, healthcare was practiced largely in the home. Early American hospitals closely resembled hospices; you didn't go to one to get well, you went there to die, and you were segregated from others so you wouldn't infect them. People with money sought treatment directly from physicians, but because true medicine was still largely undiscovered, the "cures" of the day were just as likely to kill. For example, George Washington was famously bled with leeches, the prescribed cure for "bad blood," which hastened, rather than forestalled, his death from pneumonia.

The first true healthcare facilities were drug stores, which became popular in the nineteenth century. Similar to today's pharmacies, drug stores emphasized wellness products and drugs — some of which, like the medical procedures of the day, caused more harm than good. They also fostered a sense of community and health awareness.

Long before any other segment of the healthcare industry did so, drug stores recognized that consumers had innate desires to maintain, if not improve, their states of wellness. Charles Walgreen, founder of the pharmacy chain that still bears his name, was the first to modernize and franchise his drug stores, spreading the incipient wellness industry across the country and establishing a retail market that has since been emulated by scores of other chains.

The healthcare system existed as such for a century and a half. Physicians and hospitals treated acute illness and injuries, drug stores dispensed medicine and wellness products, and consumers mostly remained ignorant about their health and how to maintain it.

And now, welcome to the Information Age. Modern patients aren't content to wait for calamity to strike, nor are they willing to accept one person as the ultimate arbiter of health-related matters. And hospitals are no longer necessarily destinations of last resort; the ones that have wisely adapted to the needs of their patients know that they're in the business of keeping people well in addition to ministering to the ill and injured.

To better illustrate this paradigm shift in the healthcare industry, consider the cases of two patients experiencing cardiac problems less than three decades apart.

The first example, Patient A, had a heart attack at age forty-nine, in 1977. He was a senior executive at an American automaker and as such had great benefits. He received what any Western country would consider world-class healthcare at the time. When he had his heart attack, there were no surgical interventions, and he spent no money of his own on treatment. Nor did he make any significant modifications to his lifestyle. He and his family had limited information on the subject of heart disease and never sought a second opinion, accepting the physician's advice without question.

Patient A, in a relatively few years, succumbed to the disease.

The second example, Patient B, had a similar cardiac episode twenty-seven years later. Patient B received a stent on the night of his attack. Already fully immersed in a healthy lifestyle, Patient B didn't smoke, maintained a reasonably healthy diet and was training for a marathon at the time of his attack, which physicians determined was largely caused by genetic factors.

Patient B further responded to the cardiac episode by:

- Modifying his diet even more.

- Reading and researching his condition on the Internet.

- Participating in rehab and fitness programs.

- Actively seeking additional opinions.

In taking these steps, Patient B spent his own money — not just because he paid into his insurance program and had co-pays but because he purchased wellness products that no health insurance policy would cover, like training tapes and fitness gear.

The difference between Patient A and Patient B isn't their amount of personal commitment or a lack of desire or will to fight the problem. Each was a typical patient of his era: Patient A didn't get enough exercise or eat as well as he should have, he accepted the advice of experts because there was no alternative, and he didn't research his disease or ways to moderate its effects because no such information was easily available to laypeople. Patient A, in many ways, was the prototype of a patient.

Patient B, in contrast, was an informed, modern healthcare consumer. Like millions of Americans, he shopped for products and information to enhance his physical, emotional and spiritual health. He turned to his hospital for critical support, but he mostly relied on his own judgment when it came to routine healthcare, regularly utilizing retail America for products, information and services. Patient B represented much of the modern American public: educated, proactive and committed to wellness.

However, Patients A and B aren't mere archetypes that illustrate a point about how the healthcare industry has changed over the past thirty years. Their stories are personal and heartfelt examples of two patients who, within just one generation, clearly illustrated the transformation in healthcare consumerism.

Patient A was my father, and Patient B is my brother.

THE WELLNESS CONSUMER

My brother is a typical healthcare consumer. He understands that his health is largely his responsibility and not that of a physician he

sees once a year. He also understands that he has options for wellness treatments in addition to acute care for events like heart attacks
or other illnesses.

Americans are far more involved in making choices regarding
their healthcare than they were decades ago. This choice-driven
approach has its roots in retail, but it has progressed into all areas
of healthcare. Previously, physicians were the key decision-makers
for all aspects of healthcare, determining the services that would
be provided, the medications that would be prescribed, the hospital to which a patient would be admitted and virtually all other
aspects of a patient's care. On television, Marcus Welby, MD, was
the prototype of the caring and informed family physician. Many
real doctors fit his profile, and patients put their trust in the family
doctor's compassionate wisdom.

Today, healthcare consumers choose providers based on amenities,
quality, convenience and other traditional consumer considerations.
Twenty-five years ago expectant mothers would check into the hospital designated by their physician and stay several days to have
their babies. Today, they choose their hospitals based upon a variety of criteria including the staffing, the quality of the delivery and
recovery rooms, the instruction offered (such as lactation classes)
and the retail availability of neonatal products, to name a few.

My father lived in a *physician-centric* world where he relied upon
his physician for healthcare information, guidance and services.
Now, my brother lives — as do we all — in a *consumer-centric* world
where he makes his selections from an ever-increasing smorgas-
bord of health-related products, services and information.

Generations ago, healthcare was largely a reactive industry, and
almost everything about it was physician-prescribed. You suffered

an ailment, you went to your doctor, he prescribed a medication to treat your ailment, you filled the prescription, and you took the medication and hoped for the best. There was no second-guessing the physician, though second opinions were sometimes sought when surgery was deemed the only remaining option.

Today's wellness consumer will likely consult with a physician when something goes awry, but as a patient, his response will be assertive. A wellness consumer will research his condition and his medications, and will find an abundance of information online. He will ask questions of his physician and sometimes seek a second opinion. He believes that a doctor should communicate with him rather than expect him to blindly follow instructions. He's likely to augment prescribed medications with over-the-counter supplements.

In short, the wellness consumer wants to understand his own condition and its care, and he'll actively pursue healthful avenues for treating the condition himself.

HEALTHCARE GOES VIRTUAL

It's been said that health topics are searched for on the Internet more often than the word "sex." Google the word "diabetes," for example, and you'll receive a staggering ninety-nine million results; breast cancer gives fifty-two million listings, while heart disease gets thirty-eight million. These numbers demonstrate that there is a large market of health-information seekers on the Internet.

Rather than await physical problems, these wellness-focused consumers seek health information and strive to continually care for their own physical well-being. Wellness consumers aren't content to ignore their physical states and hope that nothing goes out of kilter, as prior generations commonly did. They actively seek a healthy balance that will preempt sickness and disease as well as the acute care that follows.

Mercola.com is a perfect example of how consumers are driving the wellness industry. The Web forum was begun by Dr. Joseph Mercola in 1997 as a place to share his newsletters. However, he eventually realized that it was an opportunity not only to recommend products but to provide them to consumers. A free site with 850,000 subscribers and 2.5 million visitors each month, Mercola.com, in a few short years, morphed from an outlet for free medical information to a retail site offering physician-recommended products. In the site's most recent update, it added a forum for providers and consumers to share healthcare-related information with each other.

Dr. Mercola wasn't a marketing genius; the market came to him because it was eager to be better informed. In fact, seventy-six percent of American consumers say they're taking action to lower their health risks and prevent disease. Just since 2000, that number has increased by more than fifty percent. Millions of Americans are seeking to live healthier, opting for the ounce of prevention to stave off the pound of cure.

Given that, medical facilities that focus on seeing sick and injured patients when they could be treating and caring for consumers aren't merely missing their portion of an enormous sector of the economy. They are also missing a core component of their mission, which is to serve the healthcare needs of the community not only by treating the acutely ill and injured but by promoting wellness. Consumers are actively and aggressively seeking assistance with their wellness and medical needs. Meeting those needs *and* remaining profitable are not mutually exclusive. In fact, they are extraordinarily complementary.

This shift from a *physician-centric* to a *consumer-centric* market system marks the rise of the healthcare consumer movement in the United States. These consumers are now the key decision-makers in the multi-trillion-dollar healthcare market. Recognizing this, successful healthcare providers will integrate reimbursed services and products with cash-and-carry retail services and products to provide the widest range of choices to their key consumers.

THE HEALTH BOOMERS

Who are these key consumers? Much of the wellness industry is driven by the Baby Boomers, the generation born roughly after World War II and before the Vietnam War. They comprise less than one-third of the population but are responsible for almost half of the economy. The Boomers are the first great consumer generation, and not only in sheer numbers. Their spending has created entire industries and their quest for lasting health is the main driver behind the consumer-wellness movement.

The Boomers have always created industries that cater to their interests and needs, from automobiles to music, movies and television. The Boomer birth rate first drove the housing market as the population in the United States soared during the '40s and '50s. Boomers then created an eager market for the home automation industry. Items that had previously been strictly luxuries or were newly invented became household necessities — including dishwashers, washing machines, refrigerators and air conditioners.

The Boomers were largely responsible for the electronics boom as well, as televisions and stereos became standard hardware for the home. The electronics boom hit another peak when Apple introduced the first home computers, and what had previously been a novelty of the modern age became a common household item, as have cell phones, iPods, BlackBerrys and global positioning systems. The personal computer, of course, led to the surge in Internet use, which subsequently led to such phenomena as the exploding volume of Internet-based retail healthcare product and services.

Healthcare will capture the attention of Boomers for the next few decades. In economic terms, it will dwarf all the previous industries the Baby Boomers have impacted. These areas of extreme retail, driven by the needs and desires of a single demographic, will continue to have profound effects on the economy.

However, the blossoming consumer wellness industry doesn't merely coincide with the aging of the Baby Boomer generation; it's being driven by it, just as Social Security and Medicare will likely be driven into bankruptcy by millions of retiring Boomers. Retail healthcare, a rapidly expanding, $500-billion market, is the first great, new retail market of the twenty-first century and the desire to remain youthful and healthy is of interest to a growing number of Americans. Wellness industries will continue to generate new products aimed at keeping us healthy and youthful, but no demographic has greater interest in or is willing to spend more money on healthcare than the Baby Boomers.

Consumer-driven healthcare has also arisen partly as a reaction to the information, products and services that have become abundant in recent years, providing consumers with choices that simply didn't exist years ago — in other words, *empowering* them to take control of their health. It's the same notion that gives employees satisfaction at work and children a feeling of independence; it gives consumers a sense that they have some control over their own well-being.

Empowered people are proactive and inquisitive. They know what they want and they know how to get it. Information has always been power, and information in the hands of the many decentralizes power. When we are all informed, we become empowered consumers, and the centralized and authoritarian holders of information and power must accommodate our needs rather than make decisions about our wellness without our participation.

Today, there are fewer passive patients than there are empowered consumers intent on participating in their own wellness. But empowerment, for all its positive effects, also has its potential problems. Autonomy without the right information can lead to bad choices, and with so many options, consumers are sometimes misled by unscrupulous purveyors. There are, of course, honest practitioners like Dr. Mercola, who provides recommendations based on what he believes is good for his patients. But there is also an abundance of advertising touting "quality" health products, the effectiveness of which is utterly unsubstantiated by fact.

Experts are needed to separate fact from fiction and useful products from unqualified competitors, and there are no better experts than healthcare providers. Who knows your medical history and what product would best serve you more than your physician?

In this arena, hospitals and physicians have opportunities to share their expertise every day. But most hospitals still operate as though they're treating patients and not cultivating consumers. Traditionally, hospitals provided acute services to their patients. If someone had a heart attack, he would be rushed to the hospital, where the latest technology would be used to save his life. Over the years, hospitals began to offer elective surgeries and optional services to expand their offerings, remain competitive and better serve their patients. Consumers gradually began to realize that they had choices, particularly when it came to services other than acute care.

In this way, hospitals discovered a well-founded adaptive strategy, but most didn't go far enough with the idea of providing services. Today's consumers want much more complete solutions to their wellness maintenance. They want a combination of services, products and information. In fact, they will even turn to outside sources when a hospital's offerings provide only a partial solution.

In this regard, the failure to build strategies around the entire patient-care continuum has left billions of dollars of potential revenue from unmet consumer needs on the table. For example, if a hospital provides radiation therapy to an oncology patient but does not include the related products and information that can enhance its effectiveness, that patient will seek out those products based upon anecdotal references from friends and family, the media and advertised offerings. They'll purchase the products elsewhere, putting money into the consumer healthcare industry and not into the hospital or its physicians. Unfortunately, this can often give the patient faith in non-recommended products of potentially dubious value.

To stem this, oncologists may recommend that their patients purchase non-metallic deodorant to use during their chemotherapy treatment because they believe that additives in traditional deodorants interfere with treatment. Clinicians can recommend certain dietary supplements and skin care products as well. However, few hospitals provide all of these services, products and information in an integrated solution; in other words, the doctor makes the recommendation but does not supply the product in addition. As a result, patients end up driving around town, seeking niche stores that provide specialty products like non-metallic deodorant. For many, their frustration is compounded by the reality that they have to discuss their newly discovered, life-threatening health conditions with a variety of non-healthcare workers employed at these stores and outlets.

A KID IN A RED SHIRT

I recently met with the CEO of a healthcare products company whom I will refer to as Charlie. He related to his own experience and frustration with incomplete solutions offered by his local hospital.

On a provider-managed weight loss program, Charlie met with the hospital's dictician as part of his regular progress review. The dietician recommended that he purchase a pedometer and a calcium supplement that she felt he needed as part of his ongoing weight management program. Of course, the hospital did not have a store that sold these products, and the dietician did not indicate specific brands or a model number for the pedometer.

Left to his own devices, Charlie visited the local Target store to complete his shopping chores. Faced with a wall filled with vitamins and a wide range of pedometers, he wasn't able to make informed choices. Left with no other options, he turned to a kid in a red shirt — a Target clerk stocking shelves nearby — for professional medical advice.

Unfortunately, the seemingly simple task of choosing the right vitamin supplement is best done with a recommendation from a healthcare professional. There are several different types of calcium supplements, each of which is absorbed into the bloodstream differently, and their resulting nutritional and health outcomes can be very different. A healthcare professional not only *can* make an informed recommendation about this supplement, but he *should* do so.

And having the recommended product readily available can simplify the process even further. Not surprisingly, you won't necessarily find the best healthcare products on the shelves of a big box store; in fact, these establishments frequently do not offer products that are the safest or the most effective. Still, this is where consumers will look when they see, for example, studies in the news that tout fish oil as good for heart health. If their healthcare providers, on the other hand, were to offer such products themselves, consumers could be assured that what they ingested matched the efficacy of the supplements used in the clinical trial.

What it comes down to is this: Do you want your medical advice coming from a kid in a red shirt? Or would you prefer an informed opinion from a trusted healthcare expert? Would you like to make second and third trips to retail establishments to locate the products your physician recommends? Or would you rather purchase them at the hospital, in your doctor's office or through your hospital's Web site before you even leave the premises? It's not just the ease of the purchase that soothes the mind in such situations; it's the knowledge that the product comes recommended by the same people with whom you trust your health.

Each day in America, millions of consumers are receiving critical health-product-related advice from incompetent sources not by choice, but because they've been given no recommendations and no better options. These are lost opportunities and lost revenue for hospitals, clinics and doctor's offices. Just as importantly, they are lost opportunities for these professional healthcare providers to serve their patients and the community as a whole.

Looking back at Charlie's situation, the proper solution to his problem would have been for the dietician to show him a sample of the specific supplement he should take. She should have explained that the hospital carried the product and that he could purchase it from her, at the on-site store or at the online store. She could have explained that the quality of the product she offered was better than what he could find in most typical retail stores, then given specific guidance on dosages, side effects and pharmaceutical interactions. She also could have demonstrated an actual pedometer and given specific instruction on its use. Like the calcium, she could have explained that the on-site store or online service had exactly the right model available — the best-quality model for Charlie's needs, readily available and at a competitive price.

In this alternate scenario, Charlie would have left his hospital with all the service, products and information he needed to comply with his weight management program. He would have had a better outcome and a far less frustrating compliance experience. Finally, the hospital would have realized a retail profit while simultaneously providing appropriate care.

That's a win-win outcome.

PATIENTS, PAYORS AND PROVIDERS

Historically, healthcare has had three primary players: the patient who receives care; the provider who provides care; and the payor, usually an insurance company, who pays the provider for services rendered to the patient. One reason why Americans have gradually become consumers is that those who pay and those who provide healthcare have changed, and patients have been forced to adapt. Though some may have liked to choose to be only patients, as in the old model of the passive recipients of institutionalized healthcare, the modern healthcare industry has virtually eliminated that option. Now, all patients are payors by default because very few have healthcare that's absolutely free.

In prior generations, people needing healthcare were strictly seen as patients, and people like my father paid none of their healthcare costs. Doctors prescribed medication, hospitals provided care, and insurance companies paid the bills. The wellness industry was limited to home remedies like aspirin and Band-Aids.

Today, however, with the shift towards health savings accounts, co-pays, deductibles and elective procedures, and with the increasing number of uninsured people, patients are also payors, constantly paying out of pocket for their own healthcare, becoming more and more directly responsible for its total cost with each passing year.

"Payor" is a term that once referred only to insurance companies, Medicare and Medicaid, but now, it should include healthcare consumers. Every time you make a co-payment or pay into your health plan, you're a payor. You're a payor when you buy vitamins or skin care products or diet books. These are health and wellness products just as much as Band-Aids and aspirin, and the average consumer is spending increasing amounts of money on just such items.

The same concept of change applies to traditional providers. Previously, people always went to healthcare professionals to be treated: doctors, nurses, hospitals, clinics, therapists and so on. Providers were the medical establishment, and they were insular. Doctors were the only ones who understood medicine, and most were reluctant or too busy to explain their decisions to mere patients.

But today, people use other means, including the Internet, books, training and consultations with physicians, to manage their own care and make their own informed decisions. Medicine is no longer an insular community because much healthcare knowledge is now available to anyone with the desire to seek it. By looking for their own solutions and following their own counsel, consumers are often their own healthcare providers.

In fact, the modern consumer is often all three of healthcare's distinct stakeholders — the patient, the payor and the provider. The positive aspect of this shift is that consumers have come to recognize that with this additional responsibility comes greater freedom to make decisions in their own best interest. Being the payor, for example, means controlling where money is spent, which lends to greater control of every outcome. For example, if the payor has a responsibility to pay for health and wellness products to supplement traditional, physician-prescribed medicine, then he also has the freedom to choose products that serve his needs.

Being a payor means more than paying into a health plan and putting out for co-pays and prescriptions. It also means making decisions about where your healthcare money goes for both reimbursed and non-reimbursed treatments. Payors, because they have greater control of how their money is spent, are in greater control of the healthcare industry than ever before. Today, being a payor means having *power*.

SOCIALLY CONSCIOUS CONSUMERS

Becoming a payor also has implications beyond the choices that benefit the individual purchaser. Healthcare consumers' retail choices can have a broader social impact.

In recent years a type of consumer has appeared who makes choices based on social responsibility *and* personal benefit. Products such as Newman's Own, which donates profits to charity, or Starbucks Ethos Water, which supports providing potable water in impoverished areas, draw consumers based on the socially responsible ways in which their proceeds are used. Thus, the socially conscious consumer adds a third party to the purchasing equation: They get a product they want or need and the company makes a profit, *and* a third party, usually a charitable organization, also benefits.

Retailers have benefited from the increasing purchasing power of socially conscious consumers and healthcare institutions are in a position to realize the same benefit. Many communities are already united around their area hospitals, organizing foundations and fundraisers to support institutions they recognize as indispensable to the well-being of the larger population. When consumers recognize that their purchasing power can support their local hospital, socially conscious economics has an effect right in their backyard.

Given this trend towards more socially aware consumerism, the pieces are in place to effect systemic change within the healthcare system. Now, what's required is the *will* to make that change.

The essential first step is that medical institutions must recognize that they are serving consumers who have free choice and a wide array of options, and thus must provide for them alternatives to competing retailers' products. Patients may not have a say in where the ambulance takes them after an accident, but they *can* choose where they purchase their health and wellness products — from any number of area retailers or from their local hospital, which supports health and wellness initiatives throughout their community. By choosing their hospital, consumers can know that they are enriching the community in which they live.

I call such socially conscious sales "mission-based retail." Again, such sales fit the definition of a perfect business arrangement: Everyone wins. The consumer has his product, the medical institution has its profit, and both are helping realize the hospital's mission, which is serving the community.

And the transition of American healthcare into a functional system has begun.

ASK THE EXPERT

An author, business school lecturer and former Fortune 500 senior executive, Harvey Hartman is a nationally recognized expert on American cultural change and the consumer activities that impact daily business products and services. Harvey has authored three marketing texts, the most recent being A Brand Called Hope: Reimagining Consumer Culture, *which explores today's consumer-driven interpretations of quality expressed through principles, values and experiences. Harvey has consulted with major pharmaceutical, food and packaged-goods companies in developing both strategic and tactical direction in today's marketplace and has consulted numerous NGO and governmental organizations, such as the EPA, the FDA, the USDA, the World Wildlife Fund, Co-op America and The Food Alliance.*

Tony: What has The Hartman Group learned in the last ten to fifteen years and what do you envision for the next ten to fifteen years relative to the healthcare IQ and behavior of the average consumer?

Harvey: I think there are a number of different consumer threads coming together. Our direction is always from the consumer perspective. These threads include things like health and wellness. The consumers continue to redefine how they want to live their lives. Health and wellness continues to be an important component of that, and it includes not just the physical aspect of it but the mental and emotional and, at times, even spiritual aspect of it. Another thread that's coming together is all about sustainability, the idea of living a better life. It's not just about us as individuals but our friends and relatives and the communities that we live in as well.

Tony: You see those two threads as linked — a person with health and wellness aspiration is also more likely to be interested in sustainability?

Harvey: Yes. The way we define this integration, which is probably the most important trend coming in the next ten years, is that consumers are actually redefining quality as the ability to live a better life for a longer period of time. As part of this redefinition of quality they're looking at better-quality life experiences. They're looking at them collectively and communally. They're looking at authentic brands, and not just in food and beverages. What's interesting is how those beliefs are acted out. It's no longer taboo that you are more involved in your healthcare and your lifestyle than ever before.

Tony: Back in the '70s it was almost considered an insult to your physician if you went for a second opinion.

Harvey: Yes, and we think the trend of seeking second opinions is a great indicator of this whole shift in culture.

Tony: Today, if you go to a typical hospital and ask about quality, they talk about an old-fashioned measurement of quality, but the consumer has a different way of measuring quality.

Harvey: When consumers traditionally talked about health and wellness, it was the traditional paradigm in which they've got to watch their weight or blood pressure and do certain things in terms of activity and eating right. But when they talk about health and wellness today, it's beyond that. Wellness is issues that you can't necessarily put a finger on. It's feeling better about yourself. It's participating in relationships with people who have similar ideals and perspective. We hear it all the time at Whole Foods Market. "It's my Whole Foods Market because they share the same beliefs that I do." So people are customizing their lifestyle. The idea of having one particular option is no longer appropriate. Whether it's a store or a hospital or a medical center, we believe that what consumers are seeking is not just one particular remedy. They're looking at a number of remedies that are most appropriate for their particular body, family and community. It's the ability to create a halo, and anything you get under this halo you feel comfortable about. At Whole Foods there's a halo of quality. People feel good about the experience and therefore the choices within that experience all meet the quality objectives.

Consumers are saying, "Help me sustain this in a meaningful way from a physical, mental and emotional aspect." It's no longer acceptable to deliver a utilitarian experience. When you deliver on service in a way that consumers feel comfortable with, using their language, using the sensory cues that are meaningful to them, they're willing to pay a higher price for these products, services and experiences. Consumers used to have everyday occasions and special occasions, but today consumers are seeking special occasions every day. And they want those special occasions and every foreseeable kind of experience that they can imagine, whether they're buying food, having dinner, or being treated.

Tony: What are your feelings on the impact of income and education levels on those trends? Most hospitals will tell you that many of the people they serve are on Medicaid and are low-income.

Harvey: What we find is that the lower income people will definitively pay premium prices for things that are meaningful to them. We find, for example, that low-income Latinos will shop at the very expensive places for good produce, meat or cheeses because those things are important to them. We also find that people believe it's better to take care of certain things upfront rather than waiting to treat it when they're ill. So let's get the best product, let's buy our kids the best coats because not only does it keep them warm, it'll keep them well so we don't have to pay bills because they're sick. So believing that lower income consumers don't have the same aspirations as high-income people is somewhat foolish.

Tony: The Internet is a great example of something consumers can participate in at a very low cost and create all kinds of new customization and personalization experiences. How do you see the shift in U.S. demographics affecting the way people view healthcare?

Harvey: I believe what we're experiencing is not necessarily assimilation but a fusion culture where we are literally creating our own culture. We don't live in the past; we just integrate those traditional elements into modern life. What we're finding in the retail arena, whether it's a large or small footprint, consumers are really seeking a place that has a unique specificity that gives it the feeling of being authentic. That's just not in services; it's in the entire experience of retail, the ability to create experiences that include both the utilitarian value of offering good quality services and the emotional connection.

Tony: Don't retail events play a key part in that process?

Harvey: Absolutely. What we believe people are looking for in retail is celebration. Let's make today a special occasion. And that's what good retailers are trying to do. Come here and let's celebrate together, if only momentarily. You can buy my brand and you can re-experience that celebration at home when you eat that brand, and it's a celebration. When we talk about reimagining culture, we're really talking about creative consumption, which is all about co-designing. And co-designing is all about consumers being involved. We find those retailers who do that well are the retailers who will have distinct competitive advantages long-term.

Tony: It feels like the health and wellness movement you're describing, along with the sustainability thread, is a top concern of consumers that impacts all retail. Is that the major driver in today's market?

Harvey: Yes. Nobody works in a vacuum because consumers don't buy in a vacuum. They look at things in a much broader perspective than the many sectors or categories retailers work in. You can't say, "Our sector is different," because you're not. The consumer's looking at you in a contextual way and comparing that experience with other worlds. Understanding the context of how consumers are living and shopping and using products today is incredibly important no matter what sector you're working in.

Tony: So if health and wellness is already the number-one concern, how do we foresee where those threads will take us?

Harvey: Where do we go from here? Our perspective is not necessarily to let technology drive us or let demographics drive it in isolation. Our perspective is to really understand the culture. And the more we understand how that culture is shifting, how consumers are living and shopping and using product differently, and more important, how they're seeking to redefine this quality at a higher level, be more involved in the experiences, the more we'll understand and be able to get in front of this train rather than getting on the back of it when the consumers have already passed us by.

Tony: The core healthcare industry is in absolute chaos and crisis, and it's going to get worse. At the same time, these threads and trends will continue, so the spotlight will stay on the subject. Healthcare is very modern in its techniques, but it's sort of ancient in its business practices and its definition of customer relations.

Harvey: So what's the transition? Many of the companies and industries we work in, the senior management people don't recognize that this change is no longer talked about; it's actually here and driving consumers in another way. The challenge is how to actually get there. How do I take an old infrastructure that's built on a completely different financial model than it should be built on today? How can I move faster, change what my offering is, how can I build an experience?

Tony: You see some experimentation in that area. For example, Wal-Mart opened the clinics with $4 prescriptions, and suddenly the world's largest retailer is playing in the healthcare space.

Harvey: They also have the financial wherewithal to do that, but there's a company saying, "We have to go someplace else. Let's start testing options and moving in a new direction." I think the $64,000 question to many companies is, "I know I've got to be someplace else. How do I get there?" They want the road map of how to take what they have today, which is in many cases old and traditional, and transition that to a new place of where they should be. They can't do that overnight. They can't throw away those revenues that occur traditionally because they're necessary. So how do they move in a way that's seamless?

Tony: Meanwhile, consumers are moving, and healthcare systems feel they have a sacred relationship with their patients, but they also recognize the fundamentals of their business model is shifting, and they have to make this transition.

Harvey: Yes, they believe they have a sacred responsibility to their consumer, but I believe if you talk to a lot of those consumers, there's a big disconnect. It's where the customers are being touched that's affecting the disconnect, and that's fundamental with some of the infrastructure that a traditional hospital is all about.

CHAPTER 2

RETAIL HEALTHCARE ECONOMICS 101

Historically, retail consisted of the sale of goods or merchandise from brick-and-mortar stores, although recently, retail expanded exponentially with the advent of the Internet. Retail healthcare, more specifically, was once confined to certain stores, like pharmacies and supermarkets, where health and beauty aids were sold along with over-the-counter medications. Retail healthcare was the backbone, along with prescription drugs, of the drug store industry.

Retail healthcare is, with few exceptions (most notably, prescription medications and some medical equipment like wheelchairs, canes, prosthetics and such), a cash-and-carry industry. No reimbursements and little government paperwork are required to operate most retail operations, and the business model for retail, even retail healthcare, is uncomplicated and predictable.

Conversely, the overhead for traditional healthcare is immensely complicated and the processes are so convoluted that the business model is nearly impossible to decipher. I often ask hospital administrators what a typical procedure costs: "What does it cost you to perform an appendectomy?" I'll say, and the response is usually, "We charge this much." So I'll clarify the question: "What does it actually cost, though, when you calculate staff, supplies, overhead, insurance and all the other factors that go into operating a complex system like a hospital?"

This usually ends the query, because administrators don't know the answer to that question. It's not for a lack of information; it's because there's too much information. The actual cost of a simple appendectomy — when considering the pay of each individual involved, from the surgeon, the anesthesiologist and the nurses on down to the cook in the kitchen and the custodians, as well as the overhead cost of the building, including heating and cooling, the accounts payable and receivable departments for the paperwork, insurance, property taxes, grounds maintenance and a myriad of other costs — is almost incalculable. Factor in the complicated reimbursement process and co-pays and it's no surprise that administrators can't state a specific number for a simple procedure.

Compare that to the relatively simple business of retail healthcare, particularly when the space within the facility already exists and the products have two costs: the wholesale price for which they're purchased and the retail price for which they're sold. Yes, retail also must pay salaries, overhead and taxes. But the people dispensing the products are not clinicians; they are retail staff trained to operate a retail establishment. They are not the highly paid and trained personnel required in a healthcare facility. And there's no complicated paperwork for reimbursement. Income minus expenses basically provides a bottom-line figure for profit.

The Internet further eliminates retail overhead. Retail healthcare via the Internet has no comparable element in traditional healthcare. There are medical Web sites, but no physicians are appropriately prescribing medications or performing surgeries over the Internet. Retail sales on the Internet are cash and carry (using credit or debit cards, of course) and healthcare products are no different.

CONSUMER-CENTRIC WELL CARE

Another significant difference between traditional healthcare and retail healthcare is that the latter tends to be wellness-focused while traditional healthcare is sick-care-focused. Until medical clinics, optometrists and pharmacies began to appear in conventional retail stores, retail had no ability to compete with physicians and hospitals. But because wellness care was a constantly expanding segment of the healthcare market, retail stores began adding traditional healthcare products and services to their offerings. As traditional sick-care outlets remained reluctant to explore retail opportunities, retail healthcare became an increasingly significant portion of traditional retail's base.

Because retail healthcare is often less expensive and more easily accessed than traditional healthcare, it also tends to be more consumer-focused. The positive side of this focus is that by avoiding the traditional base of information and power, consumers are able to seek out their own wellness maintenance and health options. You don't need to visit your doctor to decide which over-the-counter remedy will best treat your athlete's foot; online, there are consumer ratings of products and information on every available treatment, as well as dozens of options varying by cost, availability and efficacy.

The negative side of consumer-centric retail healthcare is that it's easy for consumers to be confused by the plethora of products available. When we rely on our own judgment to make healthcare decisions — our role as provider — we force ourselves to develop a certain amount of expertise on the subject. We can take the recommendation of the first friend we talk to, the pharmacist who fills our prescriptions or the television ad that we find amusing, but to truly make an informed decision we must first educate ourselves.

For instance, when someone is diagnosed with heart disease, he generally gets opinions from more than one doctor, seeks information from the Internet or books, and maybe joins a support group. But most of us won't go to those lengths for minor maladies. We make our own decisions which are both empowering and dangerous, as there are always charlatans offering products of little or no benefit and without our physicians' expert guidance, how can we determine the truth?

This void of information from qualified sources — our medical professionals' lack of product recommendations — is the missing sheriff in the Wild West of retail healthcare.

A DISORGANIZED MARKETPLACE

Along with a lack of professional medical qualifiers for products, the actual market is also highly fragmented and disorganized.

Consumers know which stores carry electronics, which to visit for home and garden supplies, and which ones carry clothing. And each of these established retail markets has its sub-markets: Do you want high-end electronics or something less expensive? Do you wear clothes off the rack, or do you want tailoring? Without much forethought American consumers can easily decide which retail operation is likely to have some version of the item they want for a price they're willing to pay.

Retail healthcare is far less organized, both as an industry and in the minds of consumers. It's an enormous market, but one that's comprised of tens of thousands of retailers with varying degrees of product reliability, and with few guides for consumers seeking the best available products.

Just consider some of the products and services that didn't exist or were in their infancy just two decades ago: cosmetic plastic surgery; Lasik and other corrective eye surgery; cosmetic dermatology; genetic engineering for fetus gender selection and fertility; cosmetic and reconstructive dentistry; fitness clubs and fitness equipment; pharmaceuticals for hair replacement and impotence; hormone replacement therapy; weight loss products; health food restaurants and healthy alternatives in traditional restaurants.

Who would've believed twenty years ago that McDonald's and other convenience restaurants would be serving salads and yogurt alongside their burgers and fries? Even traditionally unhealthy eateries are realizing that they're missing out on a significant segment of the consumer market if they don't offer healthy food in addition to the comfort of junk food. Along with this partial conversion to healthier options by established restaurant chains, restaurants that specialize in healthy food are booming.

Wellness-focused industries that didn't even exist twenty years ago now generate hundreds of billions of dollars of revenue. Medical spas are a good example. The National Consumers League (NCL) states that nearly ninety million Americans currently use or have used products or procedures in attempts to reduce the signs of aging. Sales of anti-aging treatments are soaring among Baby Boomers, yet, according to the NCL, fifty-three percent of women are not satisfied with the over-the-counter products currently available in their market. This dissatisfaction with packaged retail solutions has funneled more clients to spas and other alternative sources for services and treatments. As a result, the medical spa industry now exceeds $12 billion annually and is the fastest-growing segment of the total spa industry.

The goal of a medical spa is to blend the experience of traditional spa indulgence with medical-grade anti-aging treatments in one convenient location. Growth in cosmetic procedures and in the medical spa industry is expected to continue since utilization is closely tied to the anti-aging movement. Medical spas offer opportunities for hospitals, healthcare organizations and physicians, such as plastic surgeons and dermatologists, to incorporate beneficial and complementary retail-based services into their business. These businesses give hospitals access to desirable healthcare consumers with substantial disposable income.

As identified in Paul Zane Pilzer's *The Wellness Revolution*, the more affluent people become, the more they're willing to spend on health and wellness in all its forms. Finding the correct wellness product is the consumer's ultimate goal; being well is proactive, whereas treating illness and disease is reactive, and those seeking wellness will make every effort to find the solution that fits them best.

In a few years, Generation X — those born between 1965 and 1983 — will reach mid-life. This generation was raised with a better grasp of nutrition than their parents; they were the first children raised with nutrition labels on food packaging and an overall awareness of health, beginning with school programs that emphasized not smoking, avoiding drugs and alcohol, and eating well. They're also computer savvy; they were the first generation to enter a workforce where computers are an essential tool rather than a novelty. Generation X will be no less wellness-focused than the Baby Boomers, and will likely have just as much disposable income to apply towards wellness.

Another factor that will drive wellness-focused healthcare will be the chronic health problems our culture is developing. The most noticeable problem already affecting Americans is obesity. Ironically, we've never known more about nutrition than we do now, yet we've never been more overweight and out of shape as a culture. A surplus of food in an affluent society has helped this trend develop, and the traditional payor-patient-provider health-care model has meant few economic ramifications for unhealthy consumers. But the system has changed, and the economics have changed, and a better focus on wellness will result.

Forty years ago, an obese individual or a chain-smoker didn't pay for poor personal choices — not with money, anyway. But as traditional healthcare continues its trend towards bankruptcy and individuals are faced with greater fiscal responsibility for their unhealthy lifestyles, obesity and smoking may decline dramatically. Remember: With power comes responsibility. A payor faced with the cost of his own healthcare decisions is more apt to follow healthy lifestyle rules than a patient with an insurance company paying all of his medical expenses.

Another factor contributing to the complexity and disorganization of wellness markets is the influence of foreign based product manufacturers and service providers. The industrialized world, which includes Europe, Pacific Rim countries and emerging economic powers like China and India, also has an interest in health maintenance. Your computer tech support is probably located in Delhi; your clothes are manufactured in Shanghai; your stocks are traded on the Hong Kong market; and with all those workers, the pool of potential healthcare consumers in other parts of the world now dwarfs that of the United States. Similarly, products — including healthcare products — from around the world are available to American consumers courtesy of the Internet, which has not only erased retail's physical walls but its borders and language barriers as well.

NUTRITONAL SUPPLEMENTS

With these open borders and retail opportunities comes, unfortunately, poorly made products and industry interference. Vitamins are a good example of a valuable product used by the majority of Americans but often distributed in poor quality and for inappropriate uses.

The value of good nutrition in preventing disease dates back hundreds of years, to before practitioners understood just what it was in food that promoted good health. Scurvy, for example, is a disease caused by deficiency of vitamin C, which leads to spongy gums and bleeding from mucous membranes, and it can be fatal. It was described by Hippocrates more than 400 years before the birth of Christ, but it wasn't until a Scottish surgeon in the British Royal Navy, James Lind, proved it could be treated with citrus fruit that British sailors began supplementing their diet with limes on long voyages.

In the United States, vitamins are manufactured according to a loose set of regulations that apply primarily to food. Few assurances regarding the purity, potency or efficacy of vitamin products are made as a result. The American Medical Association has properly recommended that adults take a multiple vitamin supplement, and countless published medical studies have exhorted the benefits of various vitamin supplements for specific conditions. Unfortunately, consumers historically couldn't purchase the vitamins used in such studies, as they are not commercially sold.

Only recently could hospitals and physicians sell vitamins that were manufactured to the specifications of those used in such studies. Companies like Care Nutrition, Inc. (www.CareNutrition.com) have developed medically-supervised, doctor-recommended nutritional support products, manufactured under strict quality controls that are now offered by hospitals and healthcare providers across the country.

Many manufacturers and distributors of vitamins are united in their fight against more stringent regulations, and they resist government attempts to reevaluate regulations and policies overseeing the manufacture and distribution of nutritional supplements. The result is that patients are essentially self-medicating with a wide range of powerful vitamin, mineral and herbal supplements that are of unpredictable quality and consistency.

Of greater concern is that there are now thousands of documented contraindications of vitamin interactions with prescribed medicines. In other words, there are probably millions of cases of patients taking vitamins that have documented interference with the prescribed drugs and clinical care that is being managed by their healthcare providers. Many of these contraindications involve serious issues in the areas of cardiology, oncology and even organ transplants.

More than 100 million Americans take vitamins every day. Over $5 billion in gross revenue goes to vitamin manufacturers generating hundreds of millions of dollars in net profits. Yes, these supplements often deliver benefits, and thus, consumers are going to continue to increase their consumption. But this is where medical professionals in hospitals need to assert their expertise by recommending quality products. Doing so ensures that patients are getting quality and appropriate products and captures the revenues for the hospitals' own operational benefits.

COSMETICS AS A HEALTHCARE PRODUCT

Another example of a product segment that has transitioned from retail into healthcare is cosmetics and skin care. Most cosmetics in the United States contain preservatives and are petroleum-based. Many studies in recent years have concluded that these preservatives and chemicals can cause cancer; the result, predictably, was the explosive growth of an organic cosmetic and skin care industry that has already reached revenue in the hundreds of millions of dollars and will eventually push the traditional industry aside.

Many healthcare providers are now educating their consumers on the potential health benefits of skin-care products that contain fewer chemicals and are organic. These providers are serving their constituencies and creating marketing opportunities for their practices. Curo Minerals (www.CuroMinerals.com) is one cosmetic product line that was designed specifically for the rigorous demands of healthcare professionals.

There are countless examples of cosmetic products designed for health-enhancing purposes that are manufactured to weak standards, sold on false promises or combined with inadequate training and information. However, many others deliver real value to consumers, which is why their overall use is increasing so dramatically. The involvement of hospitals in the sale and distribution of cosmetic healthcare products will increase their effectiveness by assuring their quality and appropriateness.

There are many retail opportunities in healthcare, each of which can help to build a stronger healthcare system by redirecting the billions of dollars that are currently flowing through traditional retail into our hospitals. The products will be better, the consumers will be healthier, and traditional healthcare institutions will be generating desperately needed revenues.

The newness of the wellness industry, the host of choices it provides and the money being spent within it can make the marketplace a very confusing arena for consumers. But there are ways to better organize the market *for* consumers while at the same time beginning to shift the economic model of today's hospitals into one of sustainability.

ASK THE EXPERT

Janet E. Porter, Ph.D., is the Executive Vice President and CFO at Dana-Farber Cancer Institute. Dr. Porter has thirty years' experience as a hospital administrator, teacher, association executive, consultant and public health leader, and has served as the Interim President and CEO of the Association of University Programs in Health Administration; the Associate Dean of Executive Education at University of North Carolina's School of Public Health; and the Vice President and COO of Children's Hospital in Columbus, Ohio, during her twelve years there. Dr. Porter has also served as a board member of the National Center for Healthcare Leadership and the Council on Linkages between Public Health Academia and Practice and the Foster G. McGaw Committee for the American Hospital Association. She currently serves on the boards of Big Sisters, Raising a Reader and Ronald McDonald House.

Tony: How is Dana-Farber responding to consumer trends and consumer involvement in healthcare?

Janet: You're probably aware that Dana-Farber is a model in terms of being patient- and family-centered. About twelve years ago, senior leadership decided we ought to do things differently and that we needed the patient's voice heard in everything we do. The best way to illustrate that is, about a year ago, I was asked to give a speech at a national meeting about a new clinical building we're constructing. It's a $350-million outpatient cancer center. People wanted to know about the planning process for that building. So I was talking about the strategic planning process, and I finished the speech, and someone came up to me and said, "It must be exhausting to work at Dana-Farber." I thought I had sounded pretty chipper. I wondered, "Why would you say that?" And she said, "Because you have to ask the patient before you do anything." And I sucked in my breath and said, "But you get it right the first time." That's just the way we do business.

There was a patient on the COO search committee when I was hired and there were patients on the building committee to select the architect. When we designed our new building, we did mock-ups of it and the architect said, "We've never changed mock-ups so many times." I asked, "Why did you change it so much? Why didn't we get it right the first time?" And he said, "It's not that you didn't get it right the first time. It's that we've never had patients and family so involved, walking through and saying, 'No, we don't think the gowning area is big enough. Where's the storage for where we throw our gowns when we're done? We don't like the lighting. Tell us about the ceiling tiles.'"

Tony: Not only did you strike a chord of consumer empowerment before the rest of industry did, but a result is that patients take an ownership in Dana-Farber in a way that they don't normally do in other hospitals or healthcare facilities.

Janet: People are in awe that the patients run this place, and that's who I work for. We have visitors from all over who comment,

"Oh, my gosh, the administrator at my hospital would never do this. They would feel so threatened." We have an advantage in our patients and staff, and we're not like a general hospital because our patients have a common traumatic experience. Cancer patients often develop an incredible passion to make things better for other cancer patients.

While I do think we're a model, I think our clarity of purpose is easier than it is at a general hospital where you've got patients who have different experiences and don't have that commonality. We shouldn't be heroes that much. There are logical reasons why it works so well here.

Tony: Not too long ago we lived in a completely physician-centered world, and patients did what their doctors told them to do. Today they still lean on their doctors, but over sixty-five percent of Americans are turning to the Internet and seeking out information on healthcare. How do you see that affecting patient involvement?

Janet: That's huge for us. Because if you're ever going to seek out who's the best and what are the choices, you're going to do it with a cancer diagnosis. You're probably not going to do that when you find out you're pregnant, or even necessarily when you need a hip replacement, but you're sure going to do it when you get a diagnosis of cancer. So the other cancer administrators at our recent national meeting were surprised to hear me say that sixty percent of our new patients are consults. Patients are coming from around the world because they feel empowered with information to make good decisions about their care. Patients are becoming ever-savvier about getting on the Web and seeking out treatments and deciding where they want to go.

Tony: How do you view traditional healthcare systems becoming more involved in patient choices as it pertains to the Internet and retail?

Janet: A friend of mine was recently diagnosed with prostate cancer on a Friday. The doctor gave him a list of Web sites and said, "I know you're not going to hear much after I tell you that you have prostate cancer. Here are a bunch of Web sites. We'll schedule a meeting with you Monday afternoon. Do your homework over the weekend and come back on Monday and we'll talk about your options." What a smart doctor. He could've sat and personally tried to educate this person for two hours and it would've been incredibly time-consuming. Instead, on Monday he met with a patient who really knew what the questions were. We still have lots to learn about how to make all the patients' retail needs easily available to them here.

Tony: On the one hand, we're encouraging people to get all the information they can get, but it sounds like sometimes they're trying to get a lifetime of education in five days, at a time when they're the most emotionally vulnerable they've ever been in their life.

Janet: A very health-savvy friend of mine recently was diagnosed with cancer of the mandible. There are two schools of thought on this woman's cancer — one is you do induction chemo, then you do surgery and you're done. Another model is to do the surgery, then do chemo and radiation afterwards. We happen to be believers in the latter, plan B. The rest of the field is mostly doing plan A. I knew this couple would get a different answer other places, and I tried to prepare them for that when they came to Farber. After our consultation, her husband sent an e-mail ten days later saying, "We've looked around and decided to go with plan A." Yet, four days later he sent another e-mail saying, "No, we've changed our minds. We're going with plan B." The point is, it's really confusing for people to think about, no matter how sophisticated and intelligent you are, because you've got stage four cancer and you're making a life-or-death decision.

Tony: The challenge is to give them information and empower them but on the other hand recognize their vulnerabilities when they're confronted by an avalanche of information.

Janet: It has been suggested that we should make videotaped consultations available to our patients. So I had a meeting with two of our disease center leaders and I'm going to try to persuade them that this is a good idea because I think there may be a lot of physician resistance. So I put this idea out and they love it. They say, "Absolutely, we should do it." In fact, one of them looked at me and said, "Janet, we recommend to the patients that they bring tape recorders, and about a third of my patients bring them." And I said, "Did it ever occur to you that we should provide those tape recorders? That our patients ought to be able to go to our gift shop and buy one, or rent one? Or what if they show up here and their tape recorder is working but their tape is broken? Can they buy a tape here?" And they said, "No." And here we think we're patient-centric, but thirty percent of our patients come with their own tape recorders and we don't feel responsible to do that for them; they've got to figure that out on their own. That's not patient-centric.

Tony: It's a point where you can use retail to enhance a patient-centric strategy.

Janet: Yes, that's an excellent way to say it.

Tony: What's next in the world of the consumer in the cancer care world? You've already got a pretty high level of consumer involvement. Where do you go from here?

Janet: There's a lot of talk about patients having portable medical records, having a credit card that potentially has their medical record on it. If we could somehow condense the patient's information onto something they could automatically swipe or have added to, wouldn't it be nice? Rather than a piece of paper, we think about it in a computer as a written document where we've written pharmacy orders, lab tests and physician consultations. Potentially, if the medical record was instead a video medical record, think about the end-patient experience. I don't know that this will ever happen. But why should the patient experience or outpatient medical record be solely a written document? Why not have video? You've got a child with chronic asthma — why shouldn't that medical record that you're carrying around on a disk somewhere be a video record of all those visits with all those doctors describing the care plan and answering parental questions instead of handwritten notes?

CHAPTER 3

TURBULENT MARKET CONDITIONS

Adopting retail healthcare strategies isn't really an option for healthcare providers — it's an economic necessity. The reimbursement-based business model used by most healthcare providers was devised decades ago, and its prognosis is terminal. By adopting new strategies, traditional healthcare providers can survive.

Generations of Americans have become accustomed to the notion of retiring at age sixty-five. It's the age people retired at when Social Security was introduced by President Roosevelt in 1935, during the Depression, and it remains the retirement age today. That designated age goes back much farther than the Depression, though; it was German Premier Otto Von Bismarck who decreed sixty-five to be the age at which government pensioners could retire ... back in 1870. And the age was chosen because very few Germans lived that long.

During the Depression, reaching age sixty-five was a long-shot for most Americans, too. Life expectancy had edged up near fifty after the turn of the century, but there were no antibiotics, infant mortality was high and many women still died during childbirth. Paying for Social Security was a calculated plan. There were far more workers paying into the system than potential recipients, and it was reasoned that a retirement incentive would help seniors retire comfortably, opening up jobs for younger Americans. But there would be, it was assured, very few retirees who actually earned Social Security because most Americans would not live long enough to receive the benefit.

Social Security's sister program, Medicare, was introduced in 1965, by President Johnson, to provide health insurance for those same retired Social Security pensioners. Even in the 1960s, while life expectancy had begun creeping upward, there were still enough workers to fund both programs because there were sixteen workers for every person collecting benefits. That proportion has dwindled considerably, and is currently 3.3-to-one. By 2030 that proportion will be two-to-one.

The Baby Boomers made funding retirement easy because there were so many of them working, paying into the system to fund the retirement of their parents and grandparents. That same demographic is retiring now, and there is no equivalent workforce to pay for their retirement.

The advances of science have also confounded the notion of retirement benefits. People live far longer today than they did even forty years ago, and the cost of addressing age-related health issues grows as the population ages. That is the irony of healthcare's fiscal demise: Its efficacy has led to its downfall.

The cost of both Social Security and Medicare began to cause financial pressure as recently as the 1970s, when it became apparent that double-indexing — raising benefits at twice the rate of inflation — would quickly bankrupt the system. Today, 20.9 percent of the federal budget is allocated for Social Security, and another

20.4 percent is spent on Medicare. Healthcare, in one form or another, accounts for one out of every six dollars spent in the United States.

As problematic as funding both programs is right now, it's about to get worse. The Baby Boomers will begin retiring in a few years, and those social safety nets established generations ago will no longer be viable. The system is barely functioning now, and most likely it will be bankrupt and irreparable in less than ten years. The Congressional Budget Office has predicted that Medicare will be insolvent by the year 2019.

There are ideas about how the system might be fixed. One suggested solution is to increase the retirement age, but that's a Band-Aid for the problem, not a solution. In order to raise the retirement age to a level where there would be far fewer beneficiaries and the system would be able to sustain itself, which was the original intent of the calculation, the new retirement age would have to be ninety-two.

That's not a misprint. To have enough wage earners to sustain Medicare, the retirement age would need to be raised twenty-seven years.

If that drastic measure were not taken, Medicare would need to eliminate from consideration those retirees who don't require benefits based on personal wealth and ration care based not on need but on the viability of the proposed treatment. A final, unattractive option would be to increase the tax rate from its current 2.9 percent (which is just for Medicare) to fourteen percent.

None of these solutions have proven palatable to the public; most politicians decline to even address the issue of funding Social Security and Medicare lest they stir up a hornet's nest. Seniors become quite angry when it's suggested that benefits be amended or reduced in any way, and they're a reliable voting block on such issues. But clearly, the current funding system has nearly been exhausted.

Soon the Baby Boomers will begin retiring, and the generation that saw the greatest increase in personal wealth in American history is about to be faced with an ironic problem: Their collective retirement will likely bankrupt a system designed to protect them, and they will pass on an unprecedented economic liability to successive generations.

ECONOMIC OUTLOOK

Our current reimbursement-based system will fail. That's not a prediction but a certainty. The question is, what can be done to make healthcare profitable while maintaining its core mission of serving the needs of the community?

Healthcare costs increase the cost of every product manufactured and every service provided in this country, reducing the ability of American companies to compete in a global market. This ultimately leads to the outsourcing of jobs and the importing of products manufactured for less overseas. American companies frequently lose ground to foreign competitors who haven't been hobbled by the overhead of exorbitant insurance premiums.

It wasn't always this way. It wasn't until the late nineteenth century, a little more than a century ago, that "accident insurance" became available in the United States, first offered by the Franklin Health Assurance Company of Massachusetts. The original accident insurance operated much like today's disability insurance, intended to provide some form of support for workers who were injured at specific jobs — particularly rail and steamboat workers. The notion of insuring something like health or wellness had been suggested centuries earlier but had been deemed impractical by insurance companies, most of which were in the business of insuring tangible assets.

Before the development of medical insurance, patients were expected to pay healthcare costs out of pocket. Early medical insurance was available only to citizens who were willing to pay for their policies; industry wasn't particularly interested in keeping workers healthy. Before the creation of unions and the intervention of President Teddy Roosevelt's administration, some companies weren't particularly interested in keeping their employees *alive*.

It wasn't until the middle of the twentieth century that traditional disability insurance evolved into our modern health insurance programs. Hospital and medical expense policies were introduced during the first half of the century, and during the 1920s, some hospitals began offering services to individuals on a prepaid basis, which led to the creation of the Blue Cross organizations.

After World War II, the federal government decided to get in the healthcare business by proxy. New regulations allowed employers to list employee healthcare costs as untaxed pay, allowing companies to lower their payroll taxes. Suddenly, there was a way to compensate employees essentially off the books, and seeking benefits in addition to salary was a new employee priority because benefits weren't taxed as personal income. The healthcare industry that evolved from this landmark decision no longer survived by selling insurance one policy at a time; agents instead sold to entire companies and for the first time, corporate America had a vested interest in employee health, even if it wasn't for the most noble reason.

Initially, everyone profited from this business arrangement. But the nature of employment changed over the subsequent decades.

Working one's entire adult life for the same company became the exception, not the norm, leaving both insurers and their client companies with very little incentive to promote long-term health or wellness. Employees leaving after several years of employment wouldn't tax the healthcare policy with late-in-life medical problems; those would be someone else's problem, most likely the government's. Thus, like so many other American institutions, healthcare began to focus almost exclusively on people's immediate needs, and ignored long-term planning for the future.

The insurance and pharmaceutical industries also came to realize that there was profit to be made in creating products that provided quick-fix solutions and treatments for common problems that weren't necessarily *medical* problems. Conventional medicine in our culture has always been more focused on cures than prevention and in this case, cures were invented for conditions that weren't necessarily medical in nature.

Viagra, for example, is a prescription drug used to treat a condition that often occurs naturally in older men: erectile dysfunction. Economic realities in coming years may cause the medical establishment, government and consumers to rethink the "medical necessity" of such treatments. Although a reimbursed, insurance paid medicine today, Viagra may become a "retail" product in the future.

RISING INSURANCE COSTS

Why is health insurance so expensive? Our increased longevity is one reason. We're in the healthcare system longer and, of course, elderly people require more healthcare. A second reason is that the decline of the birth rate following the Baby Boomer generation has resulted in fewer people working and contributing to Medicare and other forms of financial support for the system. Third, patients who were once content to receive traditional healthcare treatments are now aware that wellness matters, too, and that quality of life is as important as longevity.

A recent PricewaterhouseCoopers study points to expanding utilization, created by increased consumer demand, as a cost factor. This means that consumers are seeking wellness options and the best care available, not merely the most convenient. The study also showed that new treatments and more intensive diagnostic testing have increased costs of healthcare overall. Newer treatments, medicines and tests are often more expensive than what was offered yesterday.

So, fewer payors, better and often more expensive healthcare options and an aging population are the most significant contributors to the current healthcare crisis. Even though a hospital's cost for a particular procedure may be nearly incalculable, human behavior is quite predictable. Life and health insurance are actuarial-based industries; companies can analyze certain data and predict not only how long a typical American will live but also to what disease they are most susceptible.

Some factors identified by the PricewaterhouseCoopers study that increase insurance utilization are lifestyle-related, including smoking, obesity caused by insufficient exercise and excessive unhealthy eating, excessive drinking and drug use. These are some of the same factors that increase insurance costs as well; logically, high rates of alcoholism, smoking and obesity lead to long-term health problems, which actuaries can use to predict health-related issues and life expectancy.

Private health insurance and insurance provided by employers is expensive because of all these factors, some of which are preventable. With so much federal tax money going to Medicare to treat chronic medical conditions, it's not unreasonable to expect pre-vention and wellness to take precedence, and this seismic shift will happen as economics become increasingly dire. Companies seek-ing to reduce healthcare costs already know that smoking cessation programs and nicotine patches are far less expensive than treating emphysema and lung cancer, and that regular exercise is less costly than quadruple-bypass surgery or years of Glucophage for type 2 diabetes.

In another example, *Modern Healthcare* reported in its "By the Numbers" issue (December 24, 2007) that in 2007, the cost for fighting heart disease, the nation's number-one killer, was $431.8 billion. A high percentage of heart disease is a direct result of poor diet, exercise and smoking — all issues that fall under the "well-ness" umbrella.

Equally telling was *Modern Healthcare's* statistic that in the same year, the cost of employee absenteeism just due to asthma, diabetes and hypertension — all manageable conditions — was $30.5 bil-lion. Again, people's inability or unwillingness to address wellness care leads, inevitably, to sick care. Per capita, we spent more than $7,000 on healthcare in 2007 and pharmaceutical sales were a robust $643 billion worldwide. Clearly, the cost of treating sickness rather than addressing wellness in the United States has not been as profitable for American businesses, or for the populace as a whole, as it has been for the companies that treat sickness.

Too often the prevention of illness and disease has been ignored as a partial solution to the cost of rising health insurance. However, medical institutions and the federal government need to be proac-tive in promoting wellness and healthy lifestyles. Chronic illnesses and diseases bred by poor health maintenance, treated by the healthcare industry primarily in the no-turning-back stage, are economically debilitating.

Given this, consumers must not just seek wellness programs; the public needs to demand them from healthcare purveyors, insurers and pharmaceutical companies. And the federal government needs to promote wellness rather than singularly focus on profit-driven industries to set the standards for appropriate care.

Fortunately, we see the former happening to some extent. Wellness products and treatments are constantly being introduced into the market, and though they are not covered by traditional insurance carriers, they are sought after by the public anyway. As an example, in *The Wellness Revolution*, Pilzer describes taking glucosamine, available over the counter in any pharmacy, as a treatment for osteoarthritis while debating whether to have surgery on an injured knee — a procedure that had been suggested by a number of surgeons. When he again visited one of these surgeons after taking glucosamine for one year, the surgeon asked who had operated on Pilzer's knee. When told that he had treated *himself*, the surgeon asked Pilzer not to publicize the success of the self-treatment lest it cut into his surgical business. In addition, Pilzer was astonished to learn that the surgeon hadn't even *heard* of glucosamine.

Medicine that's primarily concerned with treating illness, rather than preventing it, is losing its sway with informed consumers. These people are willing to take their business elsewhere, even to experimental or un-reimbursed remedies if the treatment will achieve what conventional sick-care cannot.

All of this market upheaval is having profound impact on hospitals. Hospitals are in a unique situation financially. Medicare chooses what it will compensate for, and how much it will pay.

Medicare frequently reduces compensation to hospitals for certain procedures and treatments; however, hospitals are still obligated to provide the services to its Medicare patients, though at additional uncompensated expense. The ever-evolving state of Medicare compensation is yet another indicator of where the reimbursement system is headed. Medicare's inevitable insolvency will continue to be seen in steadily declining reimbursement rates for procedures the hospitals are required to perform.

This is a dilemma for politicians and has become the "third rail" of American politics. Politicians are loath to cut Medicare and thus alienate older voters, but they also fear the political suicide of raising taxes and alienating all voters. Caught in this area of uncompensated or under-compensated procedures are hospitals, which will continue to be squeezed by a system by which they must abide but won't sustain them economically.

Help doesn't appear to be on the way, neither from the government nor from profit-driven industries like pharmaceutical companies and insurers. For physicians and hospitals, denying treatments isn't an option and refusing Medicare patients isn't an alternative either. One option is to actively keep people healthier and supplement traditional healthcare with a retail element.

Promoting wellness isn't only a community benefit; it's an economic benefit to the institutions that implement care. Hospitals already engender trust and provide health and wellness services and products. All they need to do to capture a share of this billion-dollar market is to engage consumers where the need is by providing products and services that promote wellness.

The flip side of the Baby Boomers' critical effect on Social Security and Medicare is their understanding of wellness as a preventive measure. Boomers are creating industries as they move through life, including medical spas, adult stem cell therapies and bio-identical hormone replacement therapies.

The effect and potential future effect on the healthcare industry of the Baby Boomer generation has been well-documented. However, their impact on creating a retail healthcare market that provides economic salvation for medical institutions will be far more positive. This may very well be the most profound result of that generation's pursuit of good health.

ASK THE EXPERT

Jim Pearson is Vice President for National Accounts, Home Care, at McKesson Medical-Surgical, a company specializing in the distribution of healthcare systems, medical supplies and pharmaceutical products. McKesson is the eighteenth-largest company in the United States and the single-largest healthcare company in the world.

Tony: McKesson was born out of a consumer healthcare movement, right? What were the early days like?

Jim: This is our one hundred seventy-fifth year in business. We reached more than $100 billion in revenue last year. We started out delivering drugs to retail drug stores with a horse-drawn buggy. From there we've grown into a *Fortune* 18 company.

Tony: What's McKesson's view of how the dynamics are changing from the consumer's perspective?

Jim: First, a lot of healthcare insurers are putting more power in the hands of the consumer. Some of the high-deductible programs want consumers more empowered and making more decisions, so a lot of the healthcare decisions are being made by the individual versus the payer or the provider. That's an area McKesson wants to be heavily involved in, to be there to provide product and services to those patients.

Tony: What changes do you see happening in health product distribution and sales?

Jim: The McKesson division I am with is in the medical products distribution business, so we distribute products to healthcare providers, mainly home-durable medical equipment providers and home health agencies, but the other area of business we're moving into is distributing to the Web-based retail provider. As we see a lot of companies moving to distribute their products over the Web, we want to be there with them.

Tony: Ten years ago distributing directly to consumers did not exist. Now you view it as strategic and something you'll build on. How many products do you have?

Jim: Ballpark, 15,000.

Tony: Is that expanding or contracting versus five years ago?

Jim: Definitely expanding. As more companies create more products to offer to home care patients, the number of products we need to be able to provide through our distribution network needs to grow.

Tony: How much of a role does insurance play in this process?

Jim: Medicare is the number-one insurer of these products. The home care providers we service deal with the major private payors, but Medicare is the big one. More providers are now looking to have more of a retail component to their business and move away from some of the Medicare and reimbursement-driven business.

Tony: McKesson must see it's important to get those options out in front of the consumers, since they're the ones making the choices. We as consumers are shopping for things…

Jim: And people are looking for information, too. A lot of consumers leave their healthcare provider with a prescription but many don't know where to go to get the product or information about it. The home care area is an ideal place to take care of a patient if you can. There's a lot of growth in home care treatment and diseases that are cared for at home that previously required hospitalization. It's more comfortable for the patient, more cost-effective, smaller risk of infection because there are fewer bad bugs than you find at a hospital. But they've got to have products and information to support their treatment. There are two things driving home health today in terms of growth: One, we're able to do more at home and two, it's an expanding market with the aging of the Baby Boomers. Plus, it's more cost-effective to treat at home versus at a hospital. A lot of insurance providers want to drive that patient into a home care setting versus a hospital.

Tony: The information area is very active. There are now tools like feedback systems where, every morning, the patient is asked a series of questions: "Are you feeling better or worse? What's your blood sugar?" etc. If all of the answers fall within the norm, nothing further happens. If they're outside of the norm, a nurse calls the patient to discuss.

Jim: It's also a benefit to the home health agency regarding the nursing shortage as well. You can reduce the number of visits necessary by utilizing this technology. There are a number of case studies that prove it's a very effective way of treating patients in their homes.

Tony: That whole movement of transferring clinical services into the home also feels like transferring the power to the consumer to manage their own healthcare.

Jim: Yes. We see that continuing, and consumers are taking charge of their healthcare and being more responsible for where their spending is going.

Tony: Are you seeing much happening in the way of online retail pharmacies?

Jim: We do a lot in the online retail pharmacy area. We provide home delivery of supplies and equipment to the country's major online retailers.

Tony: How do you think retail will ultimately have the most impact on the overall healthcare industry and its problems?

Jim: The title of our CEO's book is *Skin in the Game*[1] — you have to get patients to have skin in the game to have them be responsible and accountable for their healthcare. That's the only way to bring about change. We believe the patient can spend their money better than anyone else, and more cost-effectively than the government or a private insurer. Consumer-driven retail spending and empowerment can only improve the efficiency of the system.

CHAPTER 4

THE LONG TAIL OF HEALTHCARE

The market theory known as the "long tail" says that our culture and economy are increasingly shifting away from a focus on a relatively small number of "hits" (mainstream products and markets) at the head of the demand curve and toward a huge number of niches in the tail. In other words, a large number of products selling relatively few units each constitutes a large portion of all units sold.

As the costs of production and distribution fall, especially online, there is now less need to lump products and consumers into one-size-fits-all containers focusing on mass sales of specific products. In an era without the constraints of physical shelf space and other bottlenecks of distribution, narrowly targeted goods and services can be as economically attractive as mainstream fare.

The long tail of retail shows that low unit sales of many products contribute significantly to the bottom line. Described first in a *Wired* magazine article by editor Chris Anderson and later in his book, *The Long Tail*, the phenomenon describes how, while the million-sellers attract most of the attention, the millions of products that sell only one or two units each contribute just as much to total sales revenue.[1] At the head of a demand curve for CDs, for example, are the blockbusters, but the tail of that demand curve is incredibly long, comprised of tens of thousands of CDs, if not millions, each selling minimal amounts that incrementally accumulate to millions more sold.

The concept of the long tail is relatively new to the field of economics, and it is counterintuitive to our basic understanding of how retail works. But its effects are real, and the concept is as applicable to healthcare as it is to the sale of books or CDs or DVDs.

The traditional view of sales of a particular product is built on the belief that single products that sell millions fuel any industry's success. Take music. Million-sellers are awarded platinum album status, tracked on the *Billboard* charts and rewarded with television appearances for the band, increased concert attendance and recognition from all media. Deservedly so, because selling a million units of anything in our fragmented media culture is a noteworthy achievement.

In brick-and-mortar retail the bestseller still receives the bulk of the retail space and advertising dollars. But online, with retail space being theoretically limitless, there is room to carry and promote those thousands of products whose individual sales will create a large portion of a company's revenue. The principle facilitator of the long tail is clearly the Internet.

Books are a great example of this. Traditionally, the largest bookstores hold thousands of titles but only carry multiple copies of the bestsellers — for example, a new Stephen King book, which will sell dozens if not hundreds of copies in a single store. This premise is accepted as the retail standard. Valuable shelf and storage space can't be wasted on single copies of books that may only sell two or three copies each year, even if they are classics. The reality of conventional retail is that it's driven by the bestsellers or hits; only so much space can be reserved for "boutique" titles that may take months to sell.

The alternative to conventional retail used to be catalogue shopping. They offered a greater variety of products — but also a longer wait and shipping costs. But at least it was possible to procure products that weren't available in a store. The Sears catalogue was among the first "virtual" stores to compete with brick-and-mortar stores by simply displaying a picture of the product and shipping the item directly to the consumer (thus also bypassing warehousing and the cost of shipping to the stores). Sears realized they could reach rural consumers who had no access to their stores with their catalogue, and thus the first retailing long tail was created.

The next development in retail that led to a shorter version of the long tail was the "superstore." The book superstore was created by Barnes & Noble and carried more than 100,000 titles — more than five times the number of a conventional bookstore. By changing the physical size of a bookstore the retailer could accommodate many more titles and, consequently, many more customers. Thus appeared the next retail long tail: a large number of books contributing low individual sales to a larger whole.

But even that quickly became the old industry standard when Jeff Bezos created Amazon.com. In researching the publishing industry, Bezos saw that 1.5 million English-language books were in print at any given time, and he began to conjecture: What if all those titles were available at once, and could be sent out relatively quickly? What if there were reviews for each and easy cross-referencing for all titles? What if there were no physical boundaries at all to book retailing? What if there were no stores, just sites, and no driving, just a quick browse on the Internet? And what if the reduced overhead — no salespeople, no stockers, no building with rent and taxes and utility costs — made sales not only more convenient, but actually made buying *less* expensive than the superstore and catalogue standards? Bezos had identified a long tail market in books and established Amazon as a means to exploit that market opportunity.

Chris Anderson lists six consistent characteristics of a long tail market:

- In virtually all markets there are more niche goods than "hits."

- The cost of reaching those niches has fallen dramatically.

- Consumers must be given products that suit their specific needs and interests.

- A large number of choices flattens the sales curve; there are fewer "hits" and more productive niches, thus more cumulative sales from the long tail.

- All those niches add up to huge sales.

- With all these factors in place, the natural shape of the demand is revealed, undistorted by physical limitations, scarcity of product and distribution problems.

As Anderson explains in his *Wired* article, "A long tail is just culture unfiltered by economic scarcity."

Retail healthcare has its own demand curve long tail, and the lack of filtration created by the Internet has allowed many more products into the market — some beneficial, some of dubious value, and a few that are downright harmful. Prior to the involvement of professional healthcare providers, retail healthcare was dominated by traditional retailers who owned a share of this market for vitamins, cosmetics, home health aids and over-the-counter pharmaceuticals.

With the demand for health and wellness increasing, healthcare became an increasingly profitable retail market, but even then it was usually the domain of pharmacies, supermarkets and health food stores. Only recently have traditional healthcare providers entered the market, bringing with them high-quality products and services.

Just as the Internet created a long tail for books and music, it also created an immense variety of health and wellness products. This tail grows longer every day as it meets consumer demands. However, consumers are often confounded by misinformation and quick fixes that may not restore health or address wellness issues. Today's customer is presented with a healthcare long tail that is a mix of quality and effective products, with a smattering of fraudulent and harmful goods as well.

As long as the healthcare long tail continues to grow at an astonishing speed, provider-recommended products are the best solution for consumers. Think of diet products and how many of them "guarantee" weight loss, or diet books that promise to take the pounds off quickly. Diets are a great business, and there is no shortage of repeat customers because the vast majority of diets don't work. (Sensible portions, balanced meals and regular exercise work, but most diet book enthusiasts don't want a new lifestyle; they want an immediate solution to a long-term problem.)

The federal government acknowledges that as many as sixty percent of American adults are overweight, that type 2 diabetes is now frequently occurring in children and that heart disease is our number-one killer. And if you search Google for weight-loss products you will receive 8,390,000 results. Which one should you choose? Which one would your physician recommend? Are you getting a solution to your problem if you choose incorrectly? Could you even harm yourself if you make the wrong choice?

Many of the products on the Internet are quick fixes at best, ineffective or even harmful at worst. If even some of them were effective, obesity wouldn't be an epidemic in our country. Instead, in the Wild West of retail healthcare, there are thousands of products that claim to solve problems they have little or no possibility of actually solving.

THE NEED FOR EXPERT RECOMMENDERS

This availability of so many products and treatments, including many of dubious value, creates a need for qualified recommendations. Retail healthcare products are often unregulated, and without recommenders to serve as guides, consumers are left to purchase from manufacturers and purveyors who may sell unnecessary products and services. Some products may harm consumers, waste money and divert retail business away from companies that offer quality products and services. It is the Wild West on the Internet, and there are few guarantees of product quality or safety.

And who better to recommend quality products than healthcare providers, those to whom we entrust our health? Hospitals and physicians have access to this same long tail of commerce — the sale of a few units of many different brands. They can do it with their loyal constituency (patients who have become consumers), in a place with better foot traffic than a box retail store (hospitals, clinics and doctor's offices), using guaranteed and branded products.

One online retail service provider that is taking advantage of this model is our own Paquin Healthcare Companies (www.PaquinHealthcare.com). The company builds e-commerce partnerships with hospitals, providing turnkey solutions that include technology, products, order fulfillment and customer services. As a result, institutions can easily provide a wide range of quality products to their patients, improve patient outcomes and generate revenue, a doubly beneficial effect. This use of the Internet also creates consumers out of people who might not have an immediate need to visit the facility, or to consumers who live outside the immediate area.

As Dr. Mercola discovered with his Web site, people are not only seeking information; they're seeking products from qualified individuals. In this way, recommending a product with a hospital or physician brand is no different from prescribing a pharmaceutical or suggesting an over-the-counter medication. When a clinician recommends a product, it verifies for the patient its legitimacy and prompts him to forego lesser products that he might have chosen if left to his own devices, or with input from the aforementioned "kid in a red shirt."

When this happens, there are two main changes in the equation of retail healthcare: The profit now goes to the established and trusted healthcare provider rather than a retailer and competing manufacturer, and the patient has a better outcome as the result of using a physician-recommended product.

Physicians already make recommendations when they prescribe medications or recommend over-the-counter drugs and health aids. Placing quality healthcare products within the clinic, hospital and doctor's office, and on the institution's Web site, makes the purchase of these products serve the needs of both patients and providers.

ASK THE EXPERT

Ellen Guarnieri is the President and CEO of Robert Wood Johnson University Hospital Hamilton (RWJ Hamilton) in New Jersey, one of the nation's leading community medical centers and the only New Jersey hospital to ever receive the prestigious Malcolm Baldrige

National Quality Award from the president of the United States. Robert Wood Johnson University Hospital provides state-of-the-art care across the full range of healthcare services. In her capacity as CEO of RWJ Hamilton, Ellen is responsible for hospital operations, ambulatory care, strategic planning, new business development, medical staff development and community outreach.

Tony: How has the incredible amount of medical information available to consumers affected your business?

Ellen: Information is a powerful force; we hear this from our patients and doctors every day. Patients are going to their doctors with information soon after they print it off the Internet. We're focused on developing systems that help sort through this almost ridiculous amount of data, determining what information is most important. We recognize that we need to stay at least a full step ahead of our patients so we can guide them to the right answers for their health. There is a concept here of empowerment, giving our community members the information and support they need to make permanent lifestyle changes.

There is also an empowerment aspect of healthcare on the Internet, which includes the enabling of advanced information and knowledge retrieval, anonymity and convenience in accessing information. We have classes in community education that teach community members how to use the Internet and what sites are valid to obtain health information.

We have a very strong wellness mission here at the hospital. Last year, 150,000 people came to our education and screening programs. This population is sizeable. It expands beyond our service market, and we see a tie-in with retail healthcare as not only helping to serve the needs of those people, but another way of communicating with them and understanding how they want care, information and education delivered.

We're also seeing the need, and we're working on this in several ways, to close the link between the hospital, patient and physician.

Tony: What are some of the tactics you are employing to accomplish that?

Ellen: We're upgrading our Web site, populating it with valid, reliable health information. When a community member needs answers, they can use this resource or call our call center — the Health Connection — and a person will give them valid Web sites or connect them with an expert practitioner. The physician can clarify the information we just gave the consumer if need be, and it links that physician back to the hospital. Of course, this ties back to the personal health record, too, which is another piece we are developing.

Tony: When you Google, for example, "diabetes," you get a million results. The question is, of those million results, which ones are appropriate for me and which ones are accurate?

Ellen: People really struggle with that. Any commercial on TV that has a new product or a new medication is the latest and greatest. It drives people to their doctors demanding that product. So we hope to educate all our physicians as well, and then they can order the product online. It does complete that loop and build confidence and trust in the hospital, and that's where we really are able to do what we're supposed to do: Promote, preserve and restore the health of our community.

Tony: How do you feel about online patient health records? Many of our clients feel they are the next step in the consumer empowerment route. Of the millions of people searching online for healthcare information today, the top provider of information has only three percent of the market. Hospitals and healthcare organizations are obviously going to make a play to be information providers, and giving access to health records may be a way to do that.

Ellen: We're not intimidated about the health record because if we can establish that trust it pays off. We know that people appreciate the level of service delivery we provide, and we're very proud of our patient satisfaction scores. The community knows they'll be receiving a high level of quality, and that's important to us. Also, part of that patient satisfaction measurement we value is that we understand the patient not only in the clinical context, but that they're emotional, spiritual human beings, too.

Tony: So it's really about bringing your mission out into the community as a whole rather than waiting for them to come to you with an acute care problem.

Ellen: That's right. I was at a seminar about one year ago, and as an ice breaker to start the session, participants were asked to verbalize their organization's mission statement. After stating the mission of RWJ Hamilton, which focuses on restoring health and preserving wellness, someone commented, "Well, everybody wants that. But how do you really do that?" After several minutes of listing our programs, processes and loyalty measurements, the commenter smiled and said, "All right, we get it!"

Tony: They didn't think you knew the answer to that question.

Ellen: Right. But I let them know we do know the answer, and the programs we develop are very much focused on wellness. One of the reasons I came to Robert Wood Johnson Hamilton was because they didn't only talk wellness; they put their dollars towards the wellness initiative. So there's a pretty significant community investment from RWJ H for the communities we serve.

Ten years ago, we hired an integrative therapy nurse and put an integrative therapy program in place. Now you're starting to hear about the holistic approach to medicine, but we've been doing it for ten years. The more we give the community, the more people are interested. So as people are aging, there's that sort of look at the whole of life, your mind, your spiritual, your physical and your financial health. So we take a broad definition of what health is, and we've put resources into broadly defining the health of this community and improving it.

Tony: In 2001, fifty-one percent of Americans were proactively involved in doing wellness things on a daily basis. In 2006, that number went up to seventy-six percent. With this increased empowerment, how does that increased customer involvement impact health outcomes, in your opinion?

Ellen: Those statistics really mimic exactly what we have seen at RWJ Hamilton. Between 2001 and 2004, we have witnessed a ninety-percent increased attendance in our community education programs. In 2004, we built an 86,000-square-foot, medically-based fitness center — the RWJ Hamilton Center for Health & Wellness — to accommodate the growing number of community members eager to improve their health. We want to make sure they're doing things right.

People definitely impact our ability to deliver care because what we see now is the whole picture of healthcare financing in the United States — especially here in New Jersey, where we have a lot of unfunded care and many hospitals are struggling to provide care for people who come in so sick when they walk in the door. They consume a lot of resources in the hospital. At RWJ Hamilton, we focus on moving those resources into the wellness arena.

Tony: You've had a culture for wellness longer than most hospitals. When you started walking down this retail road, what was the response of some of the key stakeholders in the organization?

Ellen: It was met with excitement and acceptance. No small part of it was the fact we really do need to establish non-patient-revenue sources of income. So the board was particularly interested in retail, what we're calling our "alternative revenue strategy" today. Most of our board members have been part of this organization for a long time. They've been a part of this wellness mission. They were the board that won the Baldrige Award in 2004 for this hospital. So they understand the impact of doing things right, having efficient systems, learning organizations, partnering with the community and the physicians. They understand that's very powerful. New ideas aren't frightening to them. At RWJ Hamilton, we are not afraid to be first to market with a new idea.

Tony: What are some of the retail initiatives you're thinking about or have underway?

Ellen: We've already reorganized our traditional gift shop, and we're doing well there. We're starting with all the things people can see. We've remodeled our coffee shop, which is due to open soon. We have our re-engineered Web site and it's perfect timing for us; we've been working for about six months on a more robust online presence. A major segment of our Web site will be e-commerce, and we're very excited to roll out the Web site. We really do believe our patients, our community members, and our physicians want that ease, that efficiency, that kind of one-stop shopping.

We are building a marketplace here on campus. You can access it right off the lobby and we have a beautiful spot for it. The way the consultants from Paquin helped us to envision it, it's almost like the airport-style of shop with a great flow from one shop to the next. We'll have a mom and baby shop, and some other shops focused on health, life and fun. Because we also realize that if you're here and you're a visitor, sometimes you need a little respite where you can tour through the shops or bookstore or something to take a little break.

A few things we're discussing right now are, one, being able to buy prepackaged food for people who are here or who want to call and pick up a dinner. We have a wonderful chef in our café, so we're excited about exploring this right now.

We'll be rolling out our loyalty program around the same time as our Web site. We're taking some liberties with the designs we got from Paquin — making it more our own.

Tony: How many people a year do you think you come in contact with — patients, customers, community members, employees, physicians, associates?

Ellen: More than half million. We did something called the Smart Card approximately seven years ago. It was really to ease registration for services. We rolled it out at the Septemberfest, a local community event, and we had 5,000 people apply just at that one event, so we know this community will respond. They want ease and convenience, and I think they're loyal to our hospital.

Tony: How many people are in the community you serve?

Ellen: Hamilton has 90,000 residents, and that's the township where the hospital sits. Mercer County has 315,000 residents, but we actually serve six counties, so the actual number is over 750,000.

Tony: At Paquin Healthcare we're creating a library of health-care videos that will be certified by doctors. There may be a number of videos in each section and they will be used as Web-based content by our hospital clients, so people will be able to get information in a new and exciting format. We're taking this to the next level of quality standards, and we'll be working with many doctors to allow them to publish these videos. We know this will help viewers identify what Web information is credible.

Ellen: We have in place a medical advisory panel that oversees and reviews our community programs. These doctors volunteer their time to do this — not only do they go to meetings and offer their advice to us, but also bring information forward about what their patients are asking for and what their needs are. Video will be great because we already have a similar process, without video, in place.

Tony: You've said that you're trying to close the loop from a communication and understanding standpoint.

Ellen: To kick off our strategic planning initiative this year, the senior team discussed the word "university" in our name. We discussed the concept of a community-based university hospital and confirmed that it is all about continuous learning: Learning about health, learning about wellness, learning about each other. This Paquin initiative will tie in so beautifully with our mission because it really makes us the source of health information, so it goes perfectly under that university banner.

We are a learning organization. Anything the consumer needs, any health information, services, supplies, products, you're going to go to RWJ Hamilton. That's really how I'd like to position this organization over the next couple of years with the rollout of our retail strategy.

There are five hospitals in Mercer County, including a trauma center, and we have the busiest emergency department. People seek us out and we frequently know that because we already have their information. We track everyone who comes through every program with us, so we can measure our return on investment in those programs.

Tony: Some of the innovations in your ER program were precursors of the retail clinic movement, a place where you can access medical care with a certain amount of convenience. Of course, the difference is, the depth of services available far outweighs what you can get from a mini-clinic or retail clinic.

Ellen: One of the things that always impressed me about RWJ Hamilton, and the reason why I still love to come to work everyday, is the innovation and creativity. We have the opportunity to take an idea and see it from that moment of inspiration to where it actually plays out, and we continue to be energized in this way. It wasn't by luck that we received the Baldrige award. We build our programs to meet the growing and changing needs of our community; we measure success through their eyes.

Tony: How would you put all that in the context of where you are today versus ten years from now?

Ellen: We will be the leading community hospital in Mercer County. We may one day be the only one. RWJ Hamilton will be *virtually* linked to people and systems, so our service area will not be measured geographically. We'll be strongly aligned with providers for tertiary care services in order to provide that access for our community. Our retail healthcare mission will have expanded to reach people who live well outside our current service area. Wellness education will have impacted people's lifestyle choices and we will be living longer, healthier lives.

We will also have a clinically-integrated fitness center. The way this center is designed will allow patients to see what a healthy person looks like via a computer-based avatar. So you may have had a stroke or a cardiac incident, and you can view yourself healthy. People need to see what they're working toward, that there are rewards for the wellness initiatives they themselves take.

CHAPTER 5

ELECTRONIC HEALTHCARE

There are a number of technological advances that have transformed the healthcare industry in recent years. Just as payor, provider and patient roles have changed, the way healthcare is accessed and delivered has also changed. These technological advances include the Internet, electronic medical records, e-commerce, customer relationship management and personal health records. Each of these has dramatic impact on consumer-driven retail healthcare activity.

THE INTERNET

Fifty years ago, if you asked the average person what the most important invention of the past century was, the common answer would have been the automobile. What other invention changed the world so much, from the way we traveled to where we lived? Automobiles not only led to a society that increasingly ignored borders; they led to the creation of suburbs and alternate means of transporting goods — as well as to collateral issues like air pollution and traffic-related fatalities.

But ask the same question today and the obvious answer is the Internet. While the automobile made travel faster, the Internet created instantaneous and virtual travel. Nostalgic Americans recall going to the mall and the library for all of their purchases and books. No more. The telephone made communication with another individual immediate; the Internet made communication with many people instantaneous.

Physical boundaries like store size and geographic proximity are no longer relevant to Internet users: what's becoming increasingly relevant is the *number* of choices for consumers, and how best to navigate those many choices.

At first glance, the immediacy of the Internet is very inviting to retailers. No shelf space, no foot traffic, no sales staff. And because there's no physical space required, the limitless virtual space is wide open. But the competition is fierce. There are literally tens of thousands of online stores, and when utilizing search engines, what comes to the top of the list isn't necessarily the best product, or even the most cost-effective. The challenge for consumers is in deciding which one is the best.

When choosing a movie, most of us don't base our decision just on which movie sold the most tickets that week, nor do we buy a car based solely on which model sold the most that year. If personal tastes and needs are important in traditional retail purchases, surely they are just as important when researching an issue as important as one's health. Consumers need some sort of guide to help them sort out the thousands of choices with which they are faced.

This is especially true when using the Internet, where the information overload can be daunting. For instance, a Google search on "diabetes" produces 9,300,000 results. If you're a fourth grader writing a report, it's easy enough to select one of the general information sites to cull your information. But if you're a diabetic searching for more specific information on your condition, that's a lot of information to sift through. And if you're searching for products related to diabetes there won't be a shortage to choose from; the hard part will be qualifying the product from among the thousands available, particularly if you have had no guidance.

According to the Pew Internet and American Life Project, eighty percent of American Internet users have searched online for information on at least one major health topic, a number has steadily increased in the past seven years. This means that 113 million American adults use the Internet to find health information; thirty-six percent of these health seekers say that their last search was in relation to their own health situation.

As expected, younger Americans use the Internet more, but not that much more than their older counterparts. Among women from Gen-Y (ages eighteen to twenty-six), sixty percent visited a health Web site in the past year, but Gen-X women (fifty-three percent) and young Boomers (fifty-five percent) were nearly as inquisitive. Even forty-six percent of women seniors (age sixty-two and older) researched health on the Internet.

Seven percent of health seekers, or about eight million American adults, searched for information on at least one health topic on a typical day in August 2006. This places health searches at about the same level of popularity on a typical day as paying bills online, reading blogs, or using the Internet to look up a phone number or address.

Of course, some Internet browsing is just idle curiosity, but an amazing fifty-eight percent of respondents said the information they found in their last search affected a decision about how to treat an illness or condition, and fifty-five percent said the information changed their overall approach to maintaining their health. Fifty-four percent also said that the information led them to ask a doctor new questions or to get a second opinion from another doctor.

The downside to Internet use is the degree of accuracy of the information found. Many consumers report being highly concerned about the accuracy of online information. Not surprisingly, only twenty-seven percent of online consumers visited hospital sites. Again, the lack of qualified experts leaves consumers uncertain, and in some cases poorly informed.

Using the Internet is empowering for consumers and is a great resource to those with the skill and patience to navigate it. But imagine if recommended products didn't require a search engine. What if the recommendation were implied because it came from your own physician or hospital, and what if the products in question were highlighted for you in advance?

Fully one-quarter of users felt overwhelmed by the amount of information online.[1] An illness can be disconcerting enough; attempting to research it and receiving an avalanche of information may add to the frustration. So the vast number of choices, while empowering, can also be exhausting and intimidating.

The quantity of choices shouldn't be confusing or frightening. That's the real beauty of Web-based businesses: Choices can be easily identified and made readily available. The Internet is already being used in a multitude of ways by both consumers and providers to address healthcare needs of both individuals and specific population groups with identifiable health-related demographics.

People who deal with physics like to say, "Nature abhors a vacuum." I say, "Capitalism also abhors a vacuum." When the marketplace fails to meet the needs of consumers, companies will spring up to do so. To the extent that healthcare providers fail to meet the needs of retail healthcare consumers, other, less-scrupulous companies will step in to give them what they require.

CUSTOMER RELATIONSHIP MANAGEMENT

I like to ask hospital administrators who their customers are. Until a few years ago the standard answer was, "Doctors." To a certain degree, it made sense. Hospitals viewed doctors as their customers because doctors brought business to the hospital by referring all their patients to the facility. The entire hospital environment was geared towards keeping doctors happy and productive. In the late twentieth century, as long as the doctors were productive, the patients were little more than parts on an assembly line, and often felt just as welcomed.

However, that paradigm has shifted with the broadening options available to healthcare consumers. Today, most administrators are beginning to recognize that patients are their customers and should be treated as such. Yet, many of these administrators are struggling with how to see these customers as consumers seeking healthcare options in the form of both products and services. While many hospitals have reached out to their patients via Web sites with strong healthcare content, few have taken the next logical step of creating an online store where consumers can find quality, recommended products and services.

Many hospitals now are beginning to fully recognize patients, employees, physicians and the community at large as their customers. Yet few are beginning to fully implement processes within their clinical systems to engage with consumers and manage customer relationships. A common place where consumers first connect with a hospital is an emergency room visit, where customer relationship management processes are often absent.

Like most people who have children, I've had some experience with emergency rooms. A recent ER visit with my injured daughter illustrated the need for hospitals to create customer relationship management (CRM) programs, which have long been employed by many industries to automate tracking client activity and improving customer communication and service. This was a typical emergency room visit — and what typifies emergency room visits is what is wrong with the standard system.

After giving our names to the receptionist we settled into the waiting room and completed some paperwork full of questions we had answered before. We had already visited this hospital many times, and each emergency creating an opportunity for the hospital to build loyalty within my family — starting with recognizing us as their patients. Unfortunately this hospital had no method for doing this even though I had a prior relationship with the hospital; I had even been a patient there myself. I had also done business with them and supported their foundation, and even know the CEO personally.

As I sat in the waiting room, however, I realized that I could've been a donor with a wing named after me — my name still wouldn't have been recognized by the staff. All the patients in this facility were pieces on an assembly line because without a CRM program in place, the hospital viewed us all as first-time visitors, regardless of any prior relationship we had with it.

My daughter eventually saw a doctor, but while we waited, I couldn't help but think that any hospital that employs a CRM program has the opportunity to interact more intelligently with patients and have a higher rate of patient satisfaction than those facilities without a CRM system.

We've all had emergency room visits just like that one: A long wait for care interspersed with bouts of impersonal paperwork. Unfortunately, repeat visits are often the same. Not that an emergency room "frequent flyer" should get preferential treatment, but certainly, if it's your local hospital, the one where you've gone for every injury and ailment for years, the one where your children were born, shouldn't they at least recognize you when you arrive, and have a history of your needs and experiences?

A CRM program not only expedites a visit; it is also an opportunity to build loyalty. A follow-up call or a discount card for the hospital store — both potential aspects of a good CRM plan — would remind me as a consumer that this is an institution that, in addition to knowing me, also values me.

I joke that my vehicle has better maintenance records than I do, but it's true. My auto dealer keeps track of all the work that's done on my vehicle and tells me when it's time for an oil change or a tune-up. In contrast, my hospital treats me like a stranger every time I visit. Somewhere in that building, there's paperwork with my name on it, but it's not readily accessible, and particularly not in an emergency.

Instituting CRM requires some effort upfront but saves a great deal of time later. Utilizing that pile of paperwork to build a database of consumers not only helps organize information; it also appeases patients and consumers. The benefits of a CRM program are twofold:

1. The use of CRM systems creates brand loyalty. Simply put, there are choices in healthcare today. A patient who feels welcomed

and valued is more likely to utilize and ask for a specific hospital if the service recognizes them as a valued customer, rather than as another piece on the medical assembly line. No industry falters more frequently when it comes to customer service than airlines, and even they know that building loyalty, through bonus miles and upgrades, boosts business.

2. CRM systems can be used to market hospital-branded products and services both judiciously and effectively, using affordable, direct-marketing methods like email and direct mail.

A CRM program requires effort to accumulate relevant data, but the rewards to the consumer and to the hospital are tangible and substantial. Customer satisfaction may be difficult to quantify, but loyalty is reflected in retail sales, and those results *are* quantifiable.

E-COMMERCE

Each year, shopping on the Internet cuts deeper into the retail market, which was once dominated by store shopping and augmented by catalogues. Online sales will top $200 billion this year. The Internet encompasses a huge potential market that grows each year, and one that's accessible to virtually everyone with a computer.

E-commerce can also be a viable venue for traditional healthcare institutions when used to deliver high-quality products and services to consumers. Having purchased quality health products in a hospital gift shop or clinic, many consumers will seek opportunities in the future to purchase these products, without having to leave home, by way of online, e-commerce stores.

Institutions don't need to be experts in the e-commerce retail business. Such ventures can be entirely outsourced while maintaining control of the quality of the products and service. There are proactive ways to market the institution and all of its products and services online, serving the immediate community, attracting a wider e-commerce retail base and improving the institution's bottom line all at once. Paquin Healthcare Companies has developed an e-commerce solution for its hospital clients that includes thousands of products and provides all customer service (including an 800 number, email service, order fulfillment, warehousing and inventory management), essentially removing all risk associated with its operations.

One of Paquin's customers is North Shore-LIJ, a large healthcare system located in New York that added an e-commerce element to its retail strategy (www.VivoHealth.com). North Shore-LIJ is carrying products from carefully selected vendors, which helps establish added value in the form of product quality and selection. North Shore-LIJ is also using a CRM system to do permission-based marketing to their many patients, and will have more than 50,000 products available in its virtual store. Essentially, if an affiliated physician can recommend a product, North Shore-LIJ will be able to supply it, if not at its on-premises store, then online.

Fifty thousand products could be daunting to an online shopper, but North Shore-LIJ has organized its inventory by category, brand and condition/ailment. Featured categories include mom and baby, cardiology, diabetes, heart health, nutrition, orthopedics, oncology and health and wellness. There are also help centers to learn how to use the site, track orders and check account status. The site is eye-catching, modern and efficient and unlike so many of its competitors, it's all physician- and hospital-affiliated.

North Shore-LIJ has met the requirements for successfully marketing products and services online. They're selling quality products with brand names that ensure loyalty. They've made the products easy to locate and purchase at competitive prices. They're offering enough products that consumers have choices and as a result they can meet a wide range of their customers' health-related needs.

In the case of North Shore-LIJ, the hospital's primary service area will be better served by the e-commerce strategy, and there's also the prospect of capturing consumers who've never had physical contact with it before. They're one of the few hospitals to offer branded, recommended products in a sea of unknown, unqualified products.

The Internet will continue to be the Wild West when it comes to retail sales, but pacesetters like North Shore-LIJ will have the benefit of their positive reputation before they even hit that marketplace.

ELECTRONIC MEDICAL RECORDS

Choosing a new physician can be a daunting task. Finding a doctor we're comfortable with, one who is accepting new patients and who communicates with us effectively, can mean visiting a number of physicians before making a decision.

Then, there's the paperwork! Most medical records are kept on paper, and switching doctors means physically picking up one's medical records and handing them to the new doctor's staff. Most of us have never seen our records.

The vast majority of healthcare transactions and records in the United States still takes place on paper, a system that has remained unchanged since the 1950s. The healthcare industry spends only two percent of gross revenues on record keeping, which is meager compared to other information-intensive industries such as finance, which spends as much as ten percent on records. In part, it's due to the obstinacy of the established system. Change takes place slowly and often reluctantly. This transition is costly and time-consuming, and there is no clear return on investment.

Physicians would need to spend a great deal of money to update their systems to create Electronic Medical Records (EMR), and although the healthcare industry and patients might benefit, the advantage for physicians is difficult to quantify. As a result physicians have been slow to implement new EMR solutions.

But EMRs are ultimately an indispensable tool for providers, patients and insurers. Without interoperable EMRs, which can be accessed from various systems and not just internally at a healthcare institution, physicians, pharmacies and hospitals can't share patient information that is necessary for timely, patient-centered, portable care.

As an illustration, imagine that a man is found unconscious near his local hospital. If that institution uses EMRs, his records will be available to doctors even if he's never been a patient there before because the hospital will be capable of sharing records with other healthcare institutions.

Now, imagine that he's found unconscious and brought to a hospital thousands of miles from his home — fortunately, one that also has an EMR system in place. Because he can be identified, his records can be accessed in a matter of seconds. Even if he's hospitalized in another part of the world, as long as they have compatible computer software, his EMR will be accessible to his doctors.

Another benefit of the EMR system is that it allows patients to review their own records, as we are all permitted to by law. Computer access of EMRs can facilitate access to our own information — but first the healthcare industry must adjust to recordkeeping in the electronic age. EMRs are the future of healthcare recordkeeping and in the best interest of patients. Making it a priority uniformly across the healthcare industry, however, is a challenge.

This is a priority of the federal government, though industry-wide compliance is still far off. In 2004, President George W. Bush created the Office of the National Coordinator for Health Information Technology (ONC) in order to address interoperability issues and to establish a National Health Information Network (NHIN). Under the ONC, regional health information organizations have been established in many states in order to promote the sharing of health information. Congress is currently working on legislation to increase funding to these and similar programs.

To attain the accessibility, efficiency, patient safety, confidentiality and cost savings promised by EMR systems, paper medical records must be incorporated into patients' records. Scanning these records to an EMR is expensive and time-consuming, and must be done carefully to ensure exact capture of the content.

But the future of medical records is digital entries in a computer. It may be necessary to scan existing paper records, and that may be difficult, but the goal, going forward, should be to make every record digital.

As with any medical information, with EMRs, privacy is of course a concern. According to the *Los Angeles Times*, roughly 150 people (from doctors and nurses to technicians and billing clerks) have access to at least part of a patient's records during a hospitalization, and 600,000 payors, providers and other entities that handle providers' billing data have some access.[2] Interlocking this database across the United States, and worldwide, will create even more access points and potential patient data interception.

Creating a collaborative environment that fosters communication between physicians and information technology project managers can be difficult. Exemplifying this difficulty are several highly publicized health information technology implementation fiascos, such as one at Cedars Sinai Medical Center in Los Angeles in which physicians revolted and forced the administration to scrap a $34-million system. There are, however, several successful examples of EMR implementations in large hospitals that have had years of experience developing custom EMRs. One example is the Veterans Administration, where a system known as the computerized patient record system (CPRS) allows healthcare providers to review and update a patient's electronic medical record at any of the VA's more than 1,000 facilities. CPRS also includes the ability to place orders for medications, special procedures, X-rays, patient care, nursing, diets and laboratory tests.

Great Britain's National Health Service (NHS) has a goal of creating centralized EMRs for 60 million patients by 2010, but that quest is facilitated by an existing social medicine construct. The sooner America's healthcare systems can afford to create a similar EMR objective, the sooner our archaic paper recordkeeping can be shelved permanently.

Hospitals and doctors, having been introduced to the Consumer Age, will adjust to the Electronic Age. Those with the best services, the best facilities and the best products will have an economic advantage over institutions that remain solidly in the business of physician-centric sick-care.

The ability of hospitals to identify and meet the needs of their patient population will be revolutionized by the adoption of EMR systems. Ultimately, EMR systems will integrate with the CRMs discussed previously.

PERSONAL HEALTH RECORDS

In addition to EMRs, consumers are also taking the initiative to store their own records so they can make them available to hospitals or physicians as they deem necessary, and to make them easily transferable. Such records are known as Personal Health Records (PHRs).

If access to one's EMR is empowering, then the advent of PHRs is expected to be more so, as well as a means for bringing healthcare costs under control. And PHRs, unlike EMRs, are designed solely for the consumer, with information not merely represented but packaged to suggest trends and healthful lifestyles.

If you're one of the few Americans whose doctor or hospital has created an EMR for you, then your medical information is already conveniently packaged and accessible. But if your employer has created a PHR database, then your records are available to you or to healthcare providers with whom you wish to share them.

Some large companies are starting to recognize the value of PHRs because organized and accessible health information improves individual health and potentially reduces costs. Internet search engine Google is introducing a PHR program with just that intent. Google Health is the company's planned health information storage program. In creating Google Health, Vice President of Engineering Adam Bosworth noted that people "need the medical information that is out there and available to be organized and made accessible to all... Health information should be easier to access and organize, especially in ways that make it as simple as possible to find the information that is most relevant to a specific patient's needs."[3]

Again, this is capitalism filling a vacuum. Despite the U.S. healthcare industry's foot-dragging, *The New York Times* estimates that about twenty percent of the population has computerized records,[4] and the Obama administration has pushed the healthcare industry to speed up the change. Google's program gives much more control to individuals — a trend that's both necessary and inevitable.

Google Health is intended to help customers make more informed decisions about their health, get personalized recommendations from specialists and share their records with others at will. It will include a health profile for medications, conditions and allergies; a personalized health guide for suggested treatments, drug interactions and diet and exercise regimens; pages for sharing information, or for receiving reminder messages to get prescription refills or visit a doctor; and pages to access directories for nearby physicians and specialists.

Just as recommenders streamline the quest for better healthcare, customized recordkeeping and personalized medical advice nicely enhance consumers' quests for better information, products and services, and enable better transfers of information to providers and insurers.

Microsoft has also entered into the health record business with the introduction of HealthVault, an online product that allows customers to store their electronic health records. The HealthVault also allows for electronic integration with home or professional medical devices. For example, you can take a blood sugar reading for your diabetes and have the information uploaded to your

HealthVault record. Healthcare providers who have been granted access to your HealthVault can then view these results as well as store their information about you there.

Rising healthcare costs have, in fact, prompted a consortium of companies to begin building federated databases to allow their 2.5 million collective employees to access their personal health records over the Internet. The consortium, which currently includes Applied Materials, BP, Intel, Pitney Bowes and Wal-Mart, expects additional companies to join soon. The healthcare records system is called Dossia, and the employers say that the net result of the system will be lower costs for employers and better healthcare for individuals.

"Employers pay about half the bills," Intel chairman Craig Barrett said of the program. "We've been AWOL in this discussion and it's impacting our competitiveness."[5] He says that Dossia could hold healthcare cost increases, which today outpace inflation by wide margins, to just about the rate of inflation.

Dossia will have, at its core, a series of databases being developed by a non-profit organization called the Omnimedix Institute. Once an employee joins the system and enters some personal information, the system will automatically supplement the data with records from outside sources like hospitals, insurance claims and physicians, so one database would house insurance claims data, another lab results and so on. Once the databases are built, the cost of adding incremental patients is expected to be pennies.

J.D. Kleinke, chairman and CEO of Omnimedix, sees the system as a means to bringing together disparate medical information systems. "Right now there is no personal medical information highway, only private toll-roads," he said. "Our goal is to build the equivalent of a highly secure, highly specialized medical Internet."[6]

The data will then come together to give patients the ability to see organized, predefined reports on their health, such as summaries of health information to take to doctor and emergency room visits, immunization histories, disease management applications and graphical representations of test results. Employees can also sync their data with mobile devices. Privacy remains a concern, so employers will have no access to the records.

The project has also garnered support from the American Academy of Pediatrics, the U.S. Department of Health and Human Services, the Centers for Disease Control and Prevention, the National Consumers League and the American Association of Family Physicians. The Dossia founders say that they hope the system will eventually expand to include many more companies and government employers.

The era of the folder stuffed with handwritten notes is finally coming to an end, and everyone with a stake in the healthcare system will eventually benefit from the transition.

ASK THE EXPERT

Paul Griffiths is the CEO of MedTouch, a company that delivers Web strategy, marketing and technology tools for hospitals and healthcare organizations to connect with patients, inform families, build trust with physicians and recruit staff. Tapping into the roles that search and social media play in health management, MedTouch develops consumer- and physician-focused marketing programs that drive volume, lower costs and address the evolving brand needs of the organization. Clients include Geisinger Medical Center, Massachusetts Eye and Ear Infirmary, IASIS, Rochester General Hospital, Southwestern Vermont Medical Center, Saints Medical Center, Brooks Rehabilitation Hospital, Culpeper PHO and many others.

Tony: What are hospitals doing differently online today to engage their customers in the community versus five or ten years ago?

Paul: Five years ago, only thirty percent of patients believed they had any input into the process of where to receive care, and what input they had was limited. Today, sixty percent believe they are *self-directing* those choices. That's a huge shift in responsibility back to the individual. Five years ago, hospital Web sites were almost entirely *explanatory* rather than experiential. Online self-service components didn't exist in healthcare. Now hospitals have realized these transactions are at the center of creating patient loyalty. Increasingly, we translate our clients' data — Web site visits, page views, path analysis and the like — into financial information. The achievement of business goals, such as driving appointments online, have become the standard language by which we communicate a Web site's effectiveness. That's an incredibly new conversation for healthcare.

Tony: What's the change in commitment you see by hospital management towards online services?

Paul: The level of commitment varies from hospital to hospital. In the most competitive parts of the country, winning consumers is paramount to growth strategy. For larger systems, the focus is much more about driving appointments strategically to the profitable, growing service lines and communicating about the comprehensive nature of those services. For community hospitals, the principal thrust is patient access, as such hospitals are required to showcase the value they bring to their community.

Online pre-registration, which reduces patient wait time, is easily manageable in a hospital of this size. However, a major issue at any size institution is that HIPAA limits the kind of conversation you can have with your own patients. As patients now feel more responsible for making care decisions, healthcare providers need to influence those decisions, and the only real way to do that is by giving patients control of that dialog while retaining the ability to measure the outcome. That kind of relationship can only happen online.

Tony: What's the next big thing for the online healthcare consumer?

Paul: Self-organization and self-referral through social media sites. Individuals with chronic diseases can now select from a variety of online support groups that didn't exist even a year or two ago. Patients from different healthcare systems can compare notes on the drugs they've been prescribed. Geography is no longer a barrier.

One recent study showed that consumers are now using social networking sites as bases for health and wellness decisions *more* than their primary care physicians. That's because, right now, it's a lot easier to get an email back from a blogger dealing with fibromyalgia than a physician. Many physicians are not permitted to use email for diagnostic conversations, so consumers are turning to each other to fill in the gaps. We hope that will change and that the hospitals that can work with these trends, rather than against them, will gain a new measure of credibility within these networks.

Tony: What about online transactions and e-commerce in terms of healthcare?

Paul: One of the biggest opportunities healthcare organizations miss is support of patients post-discharge. Since reimbursements are increasingly performance-based, healthcare providers need to ensure that patients follow through on their post-discharge responsibility. Being able to continue to provide retail service to the hospital's consumers is going to be extremely important, and one of the simplest ways to achieve that is with e-commerce.

Tony: People are establishing "homes," or virtual, trusted sites, on the Internet for every sort of service and product. How will that happen in the healthcare world?

Paul: Hospitals are overly focused on using their online presences to facilitate the back-office functions of the hospital — bill pay, for example. Once hospitals' Web sites assist patients with intake and offer healthcare delivery online, you will see these "homes" move away from the WebMDs of the world and toward the hospital sites. E-commerce creates a natural reason to return and addresses the questions every healthcare marketer struggles with — how do you build relationship with the patients of tomorrow? How do you recognize revenue from a population that has had a favorable experience with you but doesn't need your services right now?

We've worked with clients that have had working, useful patient gateways that reported on lab results and the like, but those functions don't create loyalty automatically, as was first expected. E-commerce provides a key "stickiness" component of online loyalty. You need to roll out a complete online health platform.

CHAPTER 6

PERMISSION-BASED MARKETING

One of the dangers of the digital age is how easily information can be lost; conversely, once it's on the Internet, it exists in virtual space forever.

Consumers worry about identity theft and literal theft, and as health records go, digital consumers will naturally question the security of this information as well. Will I be denied employment because my health history has been accessed? Can I be denied coverage because my pre-existing condition has been made public?

The government has the same concerns. Passed in 1996, the Health Insurance Portability and Privacy Act (HIPPA) established regulations for the use and disclosure of Protected Health Information (PHI), or any information about health status, provision of healthcare, or payment for healthcare that can be linked to an individual including any part of a patient's medical record or payment history. Hospitals and physicians may disclose PHI to facilitate treatment, payment or healthcare operations, or with authorization from the individual. However, when a covered entity discloses any PHI, it must make a reasonable effort to disclose only the minimum information required to achieve its purpose.

Thus, privacy must be maintained within the organization, and private information cannot be sold to other marketing agencies. As with any other doctor-patient interaction, the assumption of confidentiality is essential to maintaining a secure relationship with the patient.

Providers and health insurers who are required to follow this law must comply with patients' rights to access their health records, have corrections added to their health information, receive a notice that tells them how health information may be used and shared, and decide if they want to give permission before their health information can be used or shared for certain purposes, such as for marketing.

HIPPA was designed to protect consumers, but it incidentally gave them power over their own records, leading to the current push for electronic health records. It also provides individuals the discretion to allow healthcare providers to give them information and products that are of direct benefit to them. This idea, known as permission-based marketing, eliminates a great deal of time from the consumer's quest for products and services and, consequently, much of the chaff and cost from the business of marketing.

PERMISSION-BASED MARKETING

Permission-based marketing may be the most effective marketing ever invented because it utilizes consumers' permission to better target them with products and services that are of benefit to them. CRM systems are an avenue towards permission marketing and a vehicle that most consumers endorse with enthusiasm.

How do most marketers sell products? There are several traditional methods. One is interruption marketing. Unfortunately, most of us have experienced a solicitous, dinner-hour phone call, or a salesman at the door who won't take "no" for an answer. Interruption marketing has an extremely low success rate. Another marketing standard is direct-mail marketing, which also has a low response rate. Anything over two percent is considered a success. Because bulk postage is relatively inexpensive, direct-mail marketing has been, for decades, considered a viable marketing technique, and one that has aggravated potential customers far less than unexpected telephone calls.

Permission-based marketing, on the other hand, contacts consumers — in this case, patients — how and when it's most beneficial to them. All solicitations are based on the patients' healthcare needs and interests, and all contact is made with the permission of the patients.

For the hospital or clinic, gaining a patient's permission is as simple as having just one more line on a form. "Would you be interested in receiving more information from this facility/physician that is directly related to your medical condition?" Imagine if physicians had the time to personally contact each patient when a new pharmaceutical or treatment that addressed his or her individual condition was available. Imagine, as a patient, receiving reminders from your healthcare provider about office visits, information about new medications and services, and health tips.

It's as simple as the hospital asking permission to contact the patient, and as simple as the patient saying "yes." Who doesn't wish they could communicate more regularly with their doctor?

ASK THE EXPERT

Shawn Schwegman is the VP, Customer Success, for Vcommerce Corporation. In this role, Shawn is responsible for assisting

Vcommerce clients with e-commerce, marketing and growth strategies to make their businesses more successful. Shawn came to Vcommerce from Overstock.com where, as CTO from 2000 to 2005, he helped grow the company from $10 million per year in sales to more than $804 million in five short years, building Overstock's affiliate marketing as well as its books, movies, music and games departments. He also served in many other capacities including Director of Affiliate Marketing and VP of Marketing.

Tony: What is the status of healthcare transactions on the Internet today?

Shawn: Healthcare has become the single biggest application on the Internet with no end in sight. We've talked with thousands of healthcare professionals and they agree: The Internet is changing healthcare like never before. Retail healthcare is about consumers making choices in their healthcare by buying products and services, and that behavior is rapidly changing.

If you look at it from a retail perspective, we're kind of under the second or third generation of retail commerce. With the first generation, a lot of people scrambled to get online to start learning, and every retailer made a lot of mistakes in that process. I call the problem "show up and throw up." The consumer visitor would get to a retail site and be overwhelmed with static product content because the retailers throw every product at the consumer. That was sort of Web 1.0 — the beginning of e-commerce.

This went well for a lot of retailers in that boom, then growth rates in the last two years declined. There were a lot of pure-play retailers that were growing upwards of 80–110 percent year over year — eBay, Amazon, Overstock, they all had phenomenal growth. In the last two years that growth has slowed to an average of thirty to thirty-five percent.

As that growth slowed, Web 2.0 initiatives really took off. Web 2.0 is about engaging the customer and creating a customer experience above and beyond the customer showing up and buying something. That usually entails social networking, online reviews and other tools that really engage the customer. Web 2.0 is the age we're currently in, and it's all about engaging the customer and interacting with them above and beyond mere purchasing. If you look at online reviews, consumers who interact on the site above and beyond placing an order convert upwards to twenty percent higher than those who do not. That's why Web 2.0 is so important for retailers — because people realize if you engage the customer, you increase the chances of that customer purchasing something.

Tony: How do you see those consumer changes impacting what people are doing online regarding health and wellness?

Shawn: According to a 2007 Forrester report, more than eighty percent of online shoppers are researching healthcare content. Also, what's interesting is, in that research is the notion that people are becoming less brand-sensitive. It's the same thing that happened in the retail world with comparative shopping engines. I think something similar is happening in the health-care world, where people don't just take their doctor's word for it; they go out and do a lot of research online to back up whatever their doctor is telling them. Search has become such a powerful piece of our everyday lives. The word "Google" has really become a verb. People are so used to searching for information online that they're not going to just take the doctor's word — they're taking what the doctor says, then they're going online to do a lot of research to back it up.

Tony: As consumers are getting more involved in online purchasing, what's the next step consumers will take in the broad subject of retail, and specifically as it applies to health and medical products?

Shawn: Retailers are paving the way with the interactivity and forums and blogs and social mechanisms to engage those consumers. In the healthcare space there's not yet a clear victor, from an e-commerce perspective, paving the way for the oncoming tidal wave of consumer healthcare spending. Online shopping is expected to explode from around $140 billion to approximately $300 billion in the next five years.

Walgreens, CVS and Drugstore.com are selling a certain amount of traditional healthcare goods, but they're not specialty goods, they're sort of very generic, what you would find in a bricks-and-mortar drug store or grocery store. So where do consumers go who are looking online to buy? Where do they go to buy specialty types of goods like diabetes pumps or knee braces for ACL surgery and all those items that they read about or have recommended to them?

So since there's no clear leader, it paves the way for the healthcare industry to do some value-added selling. I think consumers are going to expect more and more from their hospitals and doctors. Healthcare providers are going to have to engage in e-commerce so they can provide the total solution for their customers.

Tony: The leading provider of health information on the net is WebMD, with only about four percent of the audience, so it's largely open territory right now.

Shawn: Absolutely. WebMD has a 4.15 percent market share as of April of 2008, according to Hitwise, which is a leading competitive intelligence tool. Mayo Clinic is just under two percent, and it goes down from there. There's no dominant supplier of healthcare information on the Internet. Today, there is no "home" for healthcare on the Internet, although a lot of companies are actively competing for that space. Once users find a "healthcare home" they are unlikely to change so we can see why it is so important for hospitals and local healthcare organizations to stake this territory.

Tony: With such a fragmented market, do you tell healthcare providers they can capture not only their local market but a broader market as well? Or do you think the market will remain fragmented since people have close associations with their hospitals of choice?

Shawn: In order to do that, you have to bridge the gap between content and shopping. If you look at WebMD, for example, they're really great at content, but they don't really have any commerce presence to speak of. So you've got one or the other; you either have a site to provide medical content, where people go to search for and research different health topics, but when they need to purchase something, where do they go?

Consumers don't want to bounce around to three or four different Web sites — one to look up content, one to find out what they need to purchase, and a different one to go purchase. It's time-consuming. If a single site can marry together rich medical content, an e-commerce site for purchasing healthcare goods, and a strong bond that's formed between patient and doctor, well, you've just created a powerful trifecta. If healthcare companies could pull that off, you've got, in my opinion, one of the strongest e-commerce stories in the history of e-commerce.

Tony: In healthcare, is there an opportunity for the healthcare provider to recommend products and help filter through the millions of choices?

Shawn: Absolutely, and if that happens, you have an even stronger emotional bond between the doctor and the patient. What healthcare has the potential to do from the perspective of strengthening the consumer-reseller relationship, that's every retailer's dream. If a retailer could recommend a product to a consumer and have the consumer trust them and go buy that product, that's the ultimate. You've got that in healthcare, but not many healthcare professionals are taking advantage of it.

Tony: The same goes for "trusted sites" on the Internet, the places we frequently go, like eBay, Amazon, Google, etc. So many of these sites are transaction-based, because as consumers, that's what we do. But if I go to Google and search for "diabetes," I have 3.5 million Web sites come up. How do I establish trust with any of them?

Shawn: There was a very interesting question asked that Forrester solved. When researching health topics online in the last year, how did consumers learn about Web sites or online resources used for health information? According to the study, more than seventy percent searched via Web-based search engines for that health information. More than twenty percent asked their healthcare professionals. And twenty percent asked family and friends. So they trust their family, they trust their friends and they trust their doctors, but they also search. If you can tie content with products and the know-how of a physician, you've created the perfect retail paradigm.

PATIENT-CONDITION-BASED MARKETING

Permission-based marketing saves everyone time, money and aggravation. But there's a subcategory of permission-based marketing, one that not only provides better communication between doctor and patient but specifically addresses the health issues that are most important to the patient.

Patients have implicit trust in doctors and hospitals. Witness the brusque and sometimes sloppy care many patients have received in the past because they suspended all critical judgment when it comes to the care provided by medical experts. Remember the patient leaving the hospital searching for medications and supplies because the hospital didn't supply them? He's now a consumer at a hospital that has an extensive CRM database, and he's leaving the hospital with his products in hand because his hospital has a retail healthcare component. But the interaction between provider and patient has just begun.

Here's a sample case: Imagine a patient who has had a mild heart attack, and he's recovered after visiting his local hospital, where they've not only created an EMR for him, but they've received his permission to send him information on pertinent health news. He has aftercare visits scheduled, new medications to maintain low cholesterol, and a cardiac regimen that can be maintained at the hospital's fitness center.

A week later, he receives an email reminding him of the times when the fitness classes meet. A week after that, he receives a reminder that he has an aftercare visit scheduled. Soon after comes a notice that a new, nonprescription, anti-cholesterol food supplement is available at the hospital's store, or at the virtual store if it's more convenient. It's recommended, of course, by his cardiologist, and it's institution-branded.

Our cardiac patient isn't done yet. He's just turned fifty and he's male, which means he should have regular visits for gender- and age-related conditions as well. For him, preventive screenings such as eye exams, colonoscopies and prostate exams are important to schedule at this point in his life.

His care has become interactive, topical and timely, and the short-term cost to the hospital has been easily covered by the increased retail sales and use of hospital facilities and services. As an empowered healthcare consumer, it's the best scenario possible for him, and an outcome that the hospital will repeat thousands of times.

Permission-based mailings directly benefit the patient. They're intended to improve his health as an individual, and in mass email form they're intended to further the hospital's mission of serving the healthcare needs of the community. Permission-based marketing also eliminates unnecessary contacts from the process by focusing marketing efforts on only those patients who want and need the information. Mailing cardiac information to the general populace may be somewhat helpful, but mostly it's a waste of resources. Targeting consumer needs on a person-by-person basis ensures that those who need information get it, and that those who don't need it aren't plagued with information that is irrelevant to their personal health.

In the digital age, with so much information at consumers' finger-tips, it's proactive, both as healthcare providers and as retailers, to provide information for patients without prompting and without delay. Increasingly, patients will seek out *any* information available, even though they would prefer a physician's advice.

Thus, hospitals must implement strategic marketing that provides consumers with information, services and products *before* they seek it elsewhere. Permission-based marketing can be profitable, consumer-empowering and mission-based healthcare. It is win-win retail in every facet.

CHAPTER 7

RETAIL HEALTHCARE STORES AND SERVICES

Alert companies quickly fill vacuums in services or products when consumers demand them. Healthcare is no exception. Just because the current system has reached a level of dysfunction doesn't mean there isn't money to be made. And just because traditional medical institutions have largely failed to integrate retail into their operations doesn't mean retail hasn't found a way of integrating wellness into its operations.

Established retailers have long owned a corner of the wellness industry, including the sales of health-related products available over the counter. Because these businesses already had a steady retail sales base and ample shelf space available, they carried everything from Band-Aids and sleep aids to medicated shampoo and foot massagers.

Retail's first foray into traditional medicine was the addition of pharmacy departments, which don't cut into traditional medicine's profitability and which give consumers yet another avenue for health maintenance in a retail space they already regularly visit.

But in recent years, big box retailers, grocery stores and pharmacies have begun investing in the consumer-centric portion of the industry by adding medical clinics. Such retailers now have invested in more aspects of the medical industry than most hospitals. They have healthcare professionals, nurses, pharmacists; they have prescriptions, over-the-counter products and an array of wellness products as well. Consumers who previously filled their prescriptions and bought wellness products at Wal-Mart after a medical clinic visit can now skip the first step and one-stop shop for their health products and services in one store.

Most consumers don't seek convenience first when it comes to healthcare, and they don't associate stores like Wal-Mart with healthcare. Consumers first seek quality and familiarity, two qualities hospitals and doctors provide. But in an era when many Americans lack health insurance and many emergency rooms, for the poor, have become *de facto* doctors' offices, low cost and convenience have become factors driving the establishment of convenience-care clinics like MinuteClinic, RediClinc and others.

And in terms of quality, convenience-care clinics are keeping pace with traditional healthcare. By focusing their range of services and keeping overhead to a minimum, these clinics have streamlined the diagnostic process and have made certain basics of healthcare more accessible than hospitals.

A recent poll confirms it: Conducted by *USA Today*, ABC News and the Kaiser Family Foundation, the poll found that seventeen percent of Americans reported dissatisfaction with their ability to get a doctor appointment when they need one, and twenty-five percent reported dissatisfaction with their ability to get non-emergency medical treatments without having to wait. In other words, traditional medicine is not only losing customers to retail healthcare; in some cases it's driving those patients away.

Conversely, ninety-three percent of MinuteClinic customers rate the quality of care as "excellent," and most would use the service again and recommend it to a friend or family member.

It's easy to say that many hospitals and doctors are overextended, that patients are sent away because hospitals are too few and too crowded, and that doctors are in short supply. But those are not good excuses. Hospitals close and doctors are too few partially because the healthcare industry hasn't adapted to the reality of the retail healthcare economy.

The success of retail healthcare facilities is more than indicative of the failure of the established healthcare model; it provides a model for existing healthcare institutions to better serve the public, combining consumer faith in established institutions with expanded and more accessible products and services.

So how profitable is convenient care?

By providing a cost-effective alternative to expensive and time-consuming emergency room visits, retail clinics benefit the uninsured and the underinsured and alleviate scheduling and roster pressures. Retail clinics also provide a lower-cost alternative for health plans and their members.

Modern convenient-care clinics emerged in 2000, in Minneapolis-St. Paul, with QuickMedx. By 2008, more than a dozen companies had emerged to open more than 200 clinics across the country, featuring longer hours than traditional primary-care providers, often open seven days a week and frequently located inside stores that also house pharmacies. Because their care is generally less expensive, retail clinics have quickly carved out a niche in an industry that once had a monopoly on physician care.

Since some consumers will opt for a convenience-care clinic whether it's operated in a Wal-Mart or their local hospital, the best option for hospitals, given the narrow focus, profitability and customer satisfaction associated with convenience-care clinics, is often to open their own retail clinics.

The effect would be beneficial for several reasons. Clinics often reduce emergency room crowding by providing treatments for a wide range of routine, non-urgent afflictions. More patients will be seen, including patients without insurance who will pay outside the reimbursement system. Customer satisfaction will generally increase, and profitability can result at the clinic while providing financial benefit to the hospital in the form of lower charity care and operating burden in the emergency room.

ASK THE EXPERT

Mary Kate Scott is the Principal of Scott & Company, a strategy consulting firm working with leaders of hospitals/healthcare systems, payers, medical device firms, pharmaceutical companies, retailers, technology providers and their investors to create and execute growth strategies. Her work with hospitals and healthcare systems includes creating retail strategies that also include facilitating workshops on retail clinics, new service lines, retail operations, strategic decisions and technology prioritization.

Mary Kate is an advisor to several healthcare firms and is a Director of Zounds Hearing. She serves leading not-for-profit institutions such as The Bill & Melinda Gates Foundation, California

HealthCare Foundation, GAVI Alliance, PATH and The Malaria Vaccine Initiative, and was a senior advisor with The Health Technology Center.

Tony: Why is the convenience clinic business important in the healthcare world right now?

Mary Kate: My focus is with the intersection of consumer healthcare and technology. For a long time I felt consumers would be the strongest voice in healthcare, which, until recently, was a heretical statement. The entire healthcare system has been designed around the physician. Even the payment system is not designed for the consumer, but rather the mainstream provider. What happens when the consumer really has a voice in healthcare? What will that consumer do? That answer affects everyone — hospitals, the pharmaceutical and medical device industries, insurance companies and physicians.

What we've seen over the last thirty years is consumers taking more control over their healthcare needs. Interestingly, 700 medications in the last thirty years that were once prescribed are now available over the counter. Consumers have a lot of confidence using over-the-counter meds. What we're seeing is a generation of consumers who have always been self-sufficient, and now they're making healthier decisions for themselves and their families. You'll find consumers are incredibly savvy shoppers, or if not savvy then very interested in finding options and information. And I think they're starting to approach healthcare the same way.

I'm interested in retail clinics because I think retail clinics are the first in-depth marketing opportunity for us to see what real consumers do when faced with healthcare choices that are designed for them and include spending their own money. Retail clinics are new because for the first time someone said, "I'm going to create a brand that's different and designed around you, the consumer." Most consumers prefer retail clinics because they are convenient — these clinics are located where they shop, in their own neighborhoods, and consumers respond to the ease of use. They also like to know how much they are paying and appreciate the transparency of pricing. Two-thirds of consumers use insurance plans to pay for retail clinic visits with one-third spending their own money.

How do consumers think about making different healthcare choices? There's an economic breaking point where people stop thinking of it as an alternative or a choice and say, "Okay, we have to consider making different decisions and spending our own money." I think we're on the cusp of that right now in healthcare. We've got 6.1 million people with high-deductible plans, and these people really think very differently when making healthcare choices.

This behavior will impact those with mainstream plans as deductibles increase for all plans. I spoke with a group of health insurance plan payers and asked, "Do you think the co-payments are going to hit $40, or even $60? The national average is $28." And they said, "Absolutely." It's just like the cost of gas. When gas prices rise, people respond and consider driving less or using different transportation approaches, and I think we'll see the same thing in the next three to five years in healthcare, because I believe co-payments are going to go up.

Tony: Don't retail clinics also serve an additional demographic — people who maybe wouldn't go to the doctor?

Mary Kate: Yes. they do, but the first audience they served was Gen-X moms and kids, moms twenty-five to forty with their children. They targeted a mainstream population, and they used a convenient offer. What's interesting to me is, traditional healthcare wasn't initially afraid of losing that customer segment, but I think they should have been concerned because it was interesting how easily they won over that targeted group.

Now we're seeing an expansion of the customer base. Sixty-three percent of people who visit clinics say they don't have a primary-care physician relationship. They might have access to insurance, but that doesn't mean you have access or a physician relationship. Also, we hear many people say, "I don't like the inconvenience of the doctor. I have to wait, I don't know when I'll be seen. I'd like quick, simple care."

We also see the uninsured at retail clinics. Often, if you're uninsured, you have a job that is paid by the hour. To be forced to wait an entire day to see a doctor and not get paid for a day is a hardship for many people.

Tony: Or go off hours...

Mary Kate: Going off hours, on the weekends, not having to wait is a strong proposition for the uninsured or anyone without paid time off. The other group clinics target is men. Men don't go to the doctor. Let's not kid ourselves.

Tony: That's true.

Mary Kate: Men are more likely to get their blood pressure and cholesterol checked at the dentist than at any other location. Clinics are a gender-neutral and broad age-range, friendly location. Generally, healthcare is a women-oriented industry, but polls show that going to the drug store is easy for men, convenient, but a place they go where there's a friendly nurse practitioner, not a stern, dictatorial physician. Men say, "I don't like white coats and I don't like being talked down to. I prefer to see a nurse because she listens to me and we have a conversation. I feel like I'm a partner in my healthcare decision."

When clinics first came out, other providers thought consumers would see this as a poor substitute. In fact consumers prefer this option. In some way it is reminiscent of other self-care options such as self-check-in at the airport or online; consumers like this simple option and don't see the kiosks or online as an inferior option but rather one that meets their needs.

With retail clinics what we're seeing is, for the first time, someone said, "What do consumers want? How do they want to see the pricing?" Those menus of pricing, they're so powerful because for the first time, someone talks to the consumer in their own language.

In California, a prominent, successful, high-quality primary-care physician group decided to publish their prices. They had two prices: a simple, routine visit, and a complex visit. That means something to a physician, but it's meaningless to the patient. They tried, but they're physicians and not consumer marketers. Every now and again a physician says, "I'm open after hours." And I say, "You're on the third floor of a building that doesn't get traffic past 5:00 p.m. and there's no parking after 5:00, so you're actually not accessible and it's not convenient."

Hospitals have turned into healthcare systems where they have a full suite of services, but I think we're starting to go back to specialization, even in primary-care practices. I think primary practice is going to become a specialty about managing complex, multiple-chronic-condition patients. The specialization with retail clinics and some hospitals is right care, right provider, right time. So it doesn't surprise me that hospitals are looking at retail clinics and thinking about how to integrate these service lines into their systems. In particular, hospitals that are involved in primary care, or charity care, or those faced with crowding in the emergency department.

We've also seen hospitals use retail clinics to keep patients in-network and attract new patients. They say, "I want to retain my market share, and I want to be present in consumers' lives more than the episodic way consumers use a hospital." Consumers use hospitals in more episodic ways, and a retail clinic offers an opportunity to be present in consumers' lives and connect those services with health and wellness beyond episodic conditions.

From a hospital's point of view, why include a retail clinic service line? After all, most clinics only earn about $1 million in revenue. But retail healthcare is here to stay. This is a new way for us to engage with the consumers, a way to enter the consumer market. Here's an opportunity to embark on a consumer-oriented program that is not a huge investment and that will help the hospital understand this new consumer.

MEDICAL AND WELLNESS SPAS

There are other aspects of the health and wellness industry that have grown rapidly in recent years, spurred by an interest in good health and completely separate from both traditional, reimbursement-based healthcare and physician-centric care. These services and products are essentially paid for by consumers out of pocket, confirming the role of the proactive and informed individual as the ultimate empowered consumer.

Nowhere is this more apparent than in the spa industry. The old-fashioned image of a spa is one where rest, a healthy diet and regular massages help one detoxify the body and mind. Certainly, spas still exist purely for pampering, but in the United States medical and wellness spas have emerged as a significant portion of the healthcare industry as more people seek better overall health, as well as ways to retard the aging process via holistic cures, experimental treatments and wellness regimens.

Spa consumers seek better health, as well as opportunities to reward themselves with luxurious treatments like massages, facials and nail care. No longer are mind and body considered separately when it comes to wellness care. We now know that anxiety and stress create physical illnesses, just as physical ailments can cause depression and emotional problems.

Medical and wellness spas address the wellness of the whole person, and as rest, retreat and rejuvenation have become priorities for millions who value their whole health, this enthusiasm is reflected in the booming industry that cares for such individuals. Many spas cater to specific areas of concern, such as skin care or weight control. Others combine naturalistic settings, organic diets, therapeutic massage, relaxation and other niceties as part of a package to provide customers with both a physical and a psychological break from everyday life.

While the leisure industry is generally the first to decline in earnings during an economic downturn, spa growth has remained consistent, with or ahead of leisure industry growth, for more than a decade. More than a quarter of Americans have been to a spa, and industry revenues were $9.4 billion in 2006. The largest growth in the spa industry, according to the spa industry itself, is the medical spa segment, which grew 109 percent between 2002 and 2004 while the remainder of the American spa industry grew only twenty-six percent during the same period.

Spa industry executives say there is a "revolution" in cosmetic procedures and in consumers who wish to look better without the need for cosmetic surgery. The Eastern/Asian influence continues to be very strong in the industry and there is a desire for natural as opposed to artificial products, while the trend towards medically-based products has also continued. A more recent trend in the industry is spa-influenced products such as clothing, home spas, spa like tubs and home massage tables. These are all symptoms of an industry that has chosen to adapt to consumer wants and needs.

Traditional hospitals can benefit from the boom in the spa industry as well. By including traditional spa features such as facials, massages and manicures with non-invasive cosmetic procedures, a hospital medical spa adds a wellness element that appeals to a growing segment of the population.

A medical spa, as a hospital service, can serve as the anchor of a wellness center. Services such as therapeutic massage, yoga, acupuncture, smoking cessation assistance and exercise and fitness training provide consumers with alternatives to wellness industry options that don't have the hospital affiliation and the associated reputation for integrity.

ANTI-AGING CLINICS

Related to spas are anti-aging clinics, where treatments that invigorate and heal the body mingle with regimens and products with benefits that may be dubious. Again, the Baby Boomers are driving this corner of the wellness industry, seeking ways to both feel and look better, and to slow the aging process.

The medical community once saw aging as an inevitable part of human life and didn't spend many resources attempting to slow it down or alter its effects on the body. Those with money could have had plastic surgery, but the lack of information and the field's more primitive technologies prevented consumers from seeking out therapies or products that might be of benefit.

Today, anti-aging treatments are growing and with the Baby Boomers leading the way, that investment is projected to continue growing at a record pace. Some of the procedures available at anti-aging clinics include obscure treatments like gene therapy; using electronics to excite cells, which purports to lead to healing and rejuvenation; nanotechnology; genomic research; bio-identical hormone replacement therapy; and biomarker testing of aging.

Anti-aging treatments and products can be included under the umbrella of the hospital's wellness center, again providing empowered consumers with the security of receiving services at their trusted, area hospital rather than from less credible and qualified purveyors.

CLINICALLY-INTEGRATED FITNESS CENTERS

The goal of clinically-integrated fitness centers is to promote an increase in physical activity levels in all ages and to emphasize the benefits of such a regimen. Currently, medical fitness facilities provide health and wellness programs to more than two million people in the United States, prompted by Americans seeking better health and partly because more physicians are encouraging fitness as a necessary compliment to a healthy lifestyle.

The phrase "clinically-integrated" refers to a physical fitness regimen that's designed and supervised by qualified medical personnel with the intent of balancing specific exercises with diet and nutritional supplements. The purpose of this is to address existing medical problems and prevent or slow the onset of eventual medical problems.

The aging American population has spurred the increase in the fitness center industry as a pre-emptive strike against debilitating, age-related problems. These centers, which are not to be confused with traditional gyms, focus entirely on the body's physical condition through medical supervision, clinical integration and a personal approach to program design, safety, cleanliness and customer service.

Many physicians and hospitals already provide integrated fitness regimens — at least in theory. What's missing from most of these traditional medical facilities is the equipment and supervision to perform the regimens on the premises. A hospital with a clinically-integrated fitness center has the medical professionals on staff, qualified trainers in the center, the equipment and products necessary and the reputation for serving the health needs of the community.

ASK THE EXPERT

Mark A. Nadel, FACHE, is Managing Director of Healthplex Associates, a prominent developer and manager of medically-based fitness centers as well as a fellow of the American College of Healthcare Executives. He is board-certified in healthcare adminis-tration and is the former CEO of Mercy Medical Center in Canton, Ohio. For more than fifteen years he has consulted with hospitals and health systems throughout the United States and Canada in the area of clinically-integrated medical fitness.

Tony: As a former hospital CEO, clearly you saw a need for an integrated fitness center. Describe what kind of needs you saw.

Mark: As a hospital CEO in the '80s and early '90s I was frus-trated that we talked about preventing disease and promoting health, but almost all of our resources went into treating sick-ness. As the cost for healthcare began to escalate, it became more apparent that there was a need for a different model of healthcare delivery than the traditional, acute-care hospital set-ting. I began to experiment with the concept of medically-based fitness, where patients in treatment could exercise while they were in cardiac rehab or physical therapy at the hospital or outpatient center, then continue to exercise at that location after reimbursable treatment ended.

But it was not as simple as it looked, and the business model needed to be more fully developed and defined. That led to an interest in creating a model combining ambulatory care serv-ices, physician's offices, medical fitness and retail healthcare services in a new type of facility that we call "Healthplex."

Tony: Would you consider a clinically-integrated fitness center a retail strategy because it's primarily a cash business and deals directly with patients?

Mark: Yes, but there is more to it than that. Regarding retail fitness, what works best in a healthcare setting is not a small gym with some exercise equipment but a larger and more comprehensive fitness facility that includes a variety of cardiovascular equipment, strength and resistance equipment, aerobics and general-purpose studio space, a lap swimming pool, a therapy pool and, sometimes, specialized rehab pools as well. We also find that high-quality locker rooms with steam and sauna, food service, perhaps a Starbucks and other amenities, make it more than simply a place to exercise. In order to instigate a lifestyle change with people who need to improve their health status, they have to be motivated to stick with it because exercise is boring and it hurts. So, our goal is to provide something that will keep people coming back.

Tony: Ten or fifteen years ago, how many hospitals had an integrated fitness center and where is that trend headed?

Mark: When we started helping hospitals in the early '90s, there were probably twenty-five to fifty medically-based fitness centers in the country. Today there are more than 1,000. I think that speaks to the fact that hospitals and physicians have begun to recognize that exercise is a part of the continuum of care, and a vital component to treatment of any medical condition. We don't see that trend declining at all; in fact, we see it accelerating.

Tony: What about the patients' perspective as consumers? What's their reaction?

Mark: The consumers tend to use the word "wow" a lot when they see a building that is architecturally striking, that's devoted to health as opposed to the traditional sick care, and with the retail amenities — a café, retail shops, medical spas, anti-aging centers and a high-end fitness center. It's a unique experience for the patient, which results in positive market differentiation for the sponsoring hospital.

Tony: What has your experience shown regarding hospitals' successes in building and operating these centers profitably?

Mark: As long as you're first in the market with this concept and you have accurately predicted retail fitness demand (and sized the facility accordingly), you can count on being fairly successful, and it's unlikely that competing hospitals will put a similar facility across the street. There's just too much risk for them. The other critical success factor is proper management and clinical integration of the center. This is a strategy that drives ambulatory care market share growth for hospitals if properly planned and executed.

Tony: What do you see ten or fifteen years in the future?

Mark: The model will continue to be refined but it will be an increasing factor of importance for employers. Hospitals are going to work with employers to improve employee health status with the medically-based fitness center as the core of the strategy. This is because employees who cost employers the most are the type who won't join health clubs and don't exercise. There's a need to get them into healthier lifestyles and this is a way to do it.

We'll also see hospitals shedding their fear of anything non-reimbursable or retail and embracing the opportunity to sell products and services that people need to maintain and improve their health as part of their business model. I see these retail centers and medical malls continuing to grow and expand and offer more and more products and services not covered by traditional medical reimbursement.

Tony: What's the distinguishing difference between medically-supervised fitness centers and traditional fitness centers with fitness trainers?

Mark: First, in a clinical environment a patient is following a clinical pathway. A hospital may take a patient through traditional treatment for services like cardiac rehabilitation, physical therapy and occupational medicine, and transition them from reimbursable medical treatment into a fitness center and a supervised, long-term health plan. That's something you won't find in typical gyms or YMCAs, for the most part.

A second factor is the recognition that many of the people you'll introduce to this facility are non-exercisers, have never belonged to a gym and are not likely to join one if given the opportunity. The way to attract these people is to provide medical supervision on-site, which reassures them that if they start exercising and something goes wrong, they won't be on their own.

Tony: In most of the centers you develop, membership fees are not on a long-term contract. How does that work?

Mark: In a medically integrated business model, your goal is long-term lifestyle change and health status improvement. You can't achieve that if people start and quit in a few months, which is common in health clubs. So, in Healthplex facilities, we only do month-to-month contracts and we provide incentives for our employees, not only to sell new memberships, but to keep people from quitting. As a result, our quitting rate for retail fitness members tends to be much lower than you find in commercial health clubs. That is a key factor in the medical mission.

Tony: What are some of the statistics about the improvement of people's health with fitness centers versus the problems in health without fitness?

Mark: The statistics that jump out are that people who exercise have approximately fifty percent less of a chance of developing cancer than people who don't. Heart disease occurs forty percent less with exercise. Physicians have determined that anything that gets worse with age usually gets better with exercise. It's the truism of medically-based fitness and it's why hospitals that do not provide medically-based fitness do not have a comprehensive healthcare delivery system.

RETAIL LABS

The advent of retail labs is another indicator of both consumer empowerment in choosing healthcare and the traditional industry's inability to meet contemporary consumer demands.

With retail labs, consumers can order their own blood tests to detect any number of medical problems including high cholesterol, diabetes, HIV, and Lyme disease. These retail labs don't require a physician's referral for medical tests, operating instead wholly as a retail store, and all consumers need is cash in hand.

QuestDirect, which is owned by Quest Diagnostics, is the largest diagnostic laboratory in the United States and just one of a growing number of direct-to-consumer labs that have opened in the United States in recent years. In response to this new consumer demand, a small number of existing commercial and hospital laboratories now offer testing directly to consumers without doctors' referrals. People can also buy certain at-home tests that can be mailed back to the laboratory for analysis.

This trend worries some physicians who question the medical implications of patients trying to diagnose their own conditions and interpret their own test results. They also question the legality of these direct-to-consumer laboratories, which are illegal in some states without a doctor's requisition.

But some patients use the labs not as diagnostic tools but to monitor existing conditions, and proponents of self-testing believe it gives patients more control over their health and may help in the early diagnosis of diseases. Some consumers opt for self-testing so the results don't appear on their medical records. Self-testing can also be particularly important to the uninsured, who may never seek traditional healthcare and may have diseases that would otherwise remain undiagnosed.

QuestDirect, HealthcheckUSA and many other independent laboratories encourage customers with abnormal results to see doctors, and when results are significantly out of the normal range, some labs contact consumers to advise them to see their physicians immediately.

Statistically, retail labs are more likely to be used by consumers who are healthy and insured but who, in the interest of self-monitoring, prevention and saving time, opt to have tests done independent of a physician's prescription. Because conventional labs run on physician referrals and insurance reimbursement, hospitals can augment their existing lab work (and income) by creating a strictly non-reimbursement annex or satellite lab that handles only non-referral tests, eliminating paperwork and overhead and providing a service to consumers who might be just as inclined to request blood work at a retail lab.

MEDICAL TOURISM

The National Coalition of Healthcare estimates that 500,000 people left the United States for treatments in foreign countries last year. Five hundred thousand international patients will visit India this year, infusing an estimated $2.2 billion into its economy; 200,000 patients visited Singapore in 2005 and 100,000 visited Malaysia that same year. Medical tourism is a $60-billion, global business that's growing at a rate of twenty percent a year.

At a recent presentation titled "Leveling the Global Healthcare Playing Field," Harvard Medical International president and CEO Dr. Robert Crone stated that regional health systems have achieved quality services at lower cost than American systems, global standards and benchmarks of quality are emerging, and medical tourism is growing.

Like other industries, healthcare has become a broad, competitive, global marketplace that is in direct competition with traditional American healthcare. Many foreign healthcare providers now offer services comparable in quality to American healthcare, and at less cost. Americans have shown a willingness to cross both the Canadian and Mexican borders to retrieve less-expensive prescription drugs, and there's speculation that making this activity legal may soon become a reality.

But it's the elective procedures that currently comprise the vast majority of medical tourism. For cosmetic surgery, as an example, it's smart to shop around for the best price. Empowered consumers are drawn to the international healthcare marketplace for procedures that are readily available in the United States, but for far more money than in India or Singapore.

Would most Americans fly 10,000 miles for several new dental crowns — plus a week of vacation on the beach — if they could save $1,000? A *TIME* magazine poll in May 2006 found that forty-five percent of uninsured people said they would, and nineteen percent of insured people agreed. When asked if they could save $5,000 on a procedure, sixty-one percent of the uninsured and forty percent of insured consumers answered affirmatively. Asked if they would do it if the procedure were accompanied by a vacation or business trip, even top executives with insurance said they would be more inclined to travel for their healthcare in such a situation.

Ironically, medical tourism once was almost exclusively the province of the United States, as foreigners came here for the best healthcare in the world. But U.S. healthcare no longer has that exalted rank, and since 9/11, inbound medical travel has dwindled, while outbound medical tourism from the United States is trending upward.

Medical tourism is yet another example of how, in an ever-increasingly competitive world economy, the peril of the U.S. healthcare system is being felt in ways that most consumers, and even hospital administrators, are unaware.

CHAPTER 8

THE GIFT SHOP PHENOMENON

We've all experienced shopping at a traditional hospital gift shop. You're visiting a sick or injured friend after work, and with no time to stop at the mall you arrive at the hospital empty-handed, so you hurriedly stop in the gift shop.

There you find a kind and elderly volunteer who smiles and rings up your purchase. Unfortunately, the selection is very limited and indistinct from every other hospital gift shop you've ever been in. So you grab the few remaining balloons and pay. It's the thought that counts, after all.

With the help of a success phenomenon that is unique to the hospital gift shop industry, even these poorly run, old-fashioned gift shops will outperform their mainstream retail counterparts. That is because of the pent-up demand found on most hospital campuses.

Imagine an up-to-date, more contemporary gift shop that has been remodeled to have an entirely different ambience. It's open for extended hours and features a modern look, more resembling an airport gift shop than a hospital gift shop of years past. There's a great selection and quantity of products, including not just gifts but also health- and convenience-related items. The staff is comprised of retail professionals who are knowledgeable about the products, which have the institution's brand on them to add credibility.

In this new shop you not only purchase a gift for the friend you're visiting; you also purchase a book you've been meaning to read and the vitamin supplements you've been looking for. In short, your visit is similar to a trip to an established retailer, with the comfort of institutional branding and the convenience of being located within the hospital.

Before we address the products and services such a shop would offer, let's consider the décor of the modern gift shop versus the traditional look of older stores.

Long gone are the days of white hallways, linoleum floors and fluorescent lights featured on the *Marcus Welby, MD* television show in the 1960s. Hospitals have worked to improve their facilities to respond to the desires of a changing society.

In her book, *The Substance of Style*, author Virginia Postrel explains, in compelling detail, how today's society invests in aesthetic style. She points out how the twenty-first century turned out far different than imagined by old movie directors. Gone are the ideas of high-rise, gray-concrete structures housing conformist citizens in drab clothing, eating meals in pill form for sustenance. Instead, Americans are creating their own "enticing, stimulating, diverse, and beautiful worlds," according to Postrel. People want style in their lives and they are willing to pay extra for it.

Retail is an opportunity to present a welcoming façade inside a hospital facility — something aesthetically pleasing rather than merely utilitarian. Stylish stores with trendy lighting, fashionable colors and elegant fixtures can radically change the environments of hospitals.

Florida Hospital Celebration Health, located in Celebration, Florida, is one perfect example of the use of progressive design in creating a unique and inviting atmosphere. The hospital was developed in collaboration with Disney Corporation and utilizes many of the same principles that made that company a world-class star. Visitors entering the main lobby are greeted by an atrium that is more reminiscent of a Ritz-Carlton hotel than a typical hospital.

The hospital lobby blends access to medical offices, retail stores, a health club and the hospital in a stylish, retail-like environment. Consumers feel welcomed and comfortable, and are put in a calm state that is conducive to healing — and to shopping for a wide range of products and services. Certainly, they are made to feel that such a professional facility can provide all of their healthcare products and services.

A facility like this, integrated with a progressive mission that includes retail offerings, helps the hospital completely reposition itself from a provider of acute services to a broadly defined source of everything that's health-related.

With the décor improved, let's next consider the hospital lobby you cross to reach your friend's room. This seemingly ordinary space sees more foot traffic than most retail establishments; in fact, traditional retailers consider this territory the last great, untapped retail market.

But just because potential customers are on the premises doesn't mean they're a captive audience. Each of them has become accustomed, over the years, to buying all of their health and wellness products from traditional retailers. They don't see a hospital as a viable marketplace for what they need because the hospital has never before attempted to fill that role.

In establishing a retail operation, the days of relying on volunteers and scattershot hours should be over. The customer is king. When considering retail models, consider Nordstrom, highly regarded as one of the nation's foremost companies when it comes to providing superb service to its customers. For example, the cornerstone of the Nordstrom service program is a no-questions-asked, money-back guarantee. If a customer is dissatisfied for any reason, sales associates have the authority to completely refund his or her money.

Having a first-rate retail operation in a hospital creates the opportunity to provide world class, Nordstrom-like service to the hospital's patients and consumers. In fact, hospitals should view their retail sales staff as a super-charged ambassador program that can reach out to their community and touch thousands of lives with very personal, extraordinary customer service experiences. In this situation, they're not just selling products or even brands. They're selling the hospital's integrity and value to its community.

The first step in selling the institution is in training the retail operation's staff. Before consumers can buy a product or buy into a premise, the people they buy from must be sold on the premise. In training a retail staff, everyone must be taught and continually reminded that:

- The community they serve consists of patients and would-be patients.

- All patients are potential customers.

- The customer is always right!

If a hospital's retail system generated $10 million in annual sales at an average sale of $20, they would post 500,000 sales transactions. Hospital executives need to see that as 500,000 opportunities to convey their message, one person at a time, with a level of service unprecedented in traditional healthcare.

Hospitals can provide that high level of service by helping consumers find the exact retail products they need. Earlier in the book we described a patient who, with no guidance from his healthcare provider, ran the retail gauntlet, searching for the products he needed. As a result, he was frustrated and guided by those working in traditional retail, which were under-informed. This consumer can be properly directed towards the products and services he needs, and in a hospital with a comprehensive retail plan, he doesn't even need to ask for those directions; like a prescription, they can be handed to him as he leaves the facility, with clear instructions as to where each product can be found: right on the premises, as the result of a retail healthcare strategy we call the "clinical connection."

The clinical connection is a management process driven by direct, two-way communication between the hospital clinical staff and the retail team. In a conventional store the most important piece of real estate is the dressing room, where the decision of whether or not to buy is made. In a healthcare setting, it is the clinical visit that serves that purpose.

A patient requiring any product or service should leave a clinical exam with a note indicating which products are available in the hospital store. This requires the clinical staff to be familiar with the store inventory, and the store to stock products that will be needed by patients. The clinical staff must also be aware of the services available at the hospital's retail outlets.

Hospitals are driven by a common mission to serve their patients. For instance, Summa Health System of Akron, Ohio, has the following mission statement that typifies that of many hospitals across the country:

> The mission of Summa Health System is to provide the highest-quality compassionate care to our patients and to contribute to a healthier community.

Most hospital cultures are similarly built on the premise of helping people in their communities build healthier lifestyles. A retail strategy can enhance that mission by helping the hospitals connect with their customers in times of both sickness and wellness. Healthier and more loyal customers will reward the hospitals with financial gain, allowing the institutions to provide better service to their communities.

There is a definite connection between improved patient outcomes and the use of health-related products. From the enhancement of healthy lifestyles to the more direct clinical benefits, these products are having a profound impact on millions of Americans.

Park Nicollet Health Services in Minneapolis, Minnesota, is a healthcare provider that features, among other services, a highly regarded breast cancer diagnostic and treatment center, the Jane Brattain Breast Center. Park Nicollet has recognized the need to integrate a retail product strategy into its mission and has built the Jane Brattain Boutique adjacent to their breast center. The following statement, found on their Web site, illustrates how this stylish boutique provides products as an enhancement to clinical care:

> The Jane Brattain Boutique offers women expert service and products to assist with their self-care when cancer enters their

lives. The boutique also provides caring gifts for women and their families and friends as they journey together toward health, healing and learning.

Retail outlets like the Jane Brattain Boutique are unique and therefore important market differentiators. In an industry where consumers often view competing providers as equals, hospitals must look for ways to stand out in the crowd, with additional value that is substantial and easily recognized.

The Jane Brattain Boutique is a classic example of this market advantage. The boutique is aesthetically pleasing; you can't visit the clinic without seeing it and being intrigued by its inviting atmosphere and design. Moreover, the boutique offers an important additional advantage to the clinic's patients: Visitors can buy much-needed products to support their treatments and enhance their recovery processes.

How does a hospital determine what its patients will most need? It's a developing science. Based on prior patient care records, the need for particular types of health and wellness products can be estimated. Choosing unique and name-branded healthcare products also separates the hospital gift shop from conventional retail stores. The hospital can also institute a customer loyalty program, a sort of frequent-flyer program that provides cardholders with discounts and promotional items. A loyalty program's benefits extend in all directions, providing extra incentive for consumers to use the hospital retail stores and extra income for the hospital. With an established patient database, cardholders can even be notified of discounts on products they've purchased in the past, or of products that might be of benefit to them.

The end result is a staff that is invested in the principle of providing consumers with the products they *need* (and will inevitably choose to buy *somewhere*) along with products they *desire*. Once the hospital retail operation has been implemented, the goal of the staff should be that no patient will leave the hospital campus without their health product needs fully met.

There may even come a day when, because of the combination of quality products, helpful staff and a pleasant shopping environment, patients and non-patients alike will use the hospital store as a preferred shopping destination for health and wellness products in addition to gifts, florals and convenience items.

ASK THE EXPERT

Kim Schuler is the CEO of Lori's Gifts, a hospital gift shop management firm. Kim joined Lori's in 1999, after spending a decade at Hallmark Cards, Inc. At Hallmark, Kim spent seven years in Chicago in field sales, working directly with specialty gift shops, and later in management at Hallmark's corporate office in Kansas City.

> **Tony:** What do you see happening with modern hospital gift shops?

> **Kim:** To be successful in today's competitive retail landscape, hospital gift shops must continue to evolve based on the demands of the consumer and in support of the hospital's mission. We have twenty-seven years of experience with hospital gift shops, and we currently manage 212 shops in twenty-eight states coast to coast. In the last several years we have had steady growth by opening, on average, twenty new gift shops each year exclusively in hospitals. Our hospital administrators recognize that the gift shop operation is a direct reflection of the hospi-

tal and if it's not a professionally run gift shop, then the first impression may not be positive, since the gift shop is located in the front lobby entrance.

Tony: Describe a typical gift shop. What are the kinds of products, sales volume, size and so on?

Kim: The average gift shop size is 700 square feet, although we operate locations that are as small as 200 square feet and others that are over 2,500 square feet. No two gift shops are alike. It is a collaborative effort with each hospital partner to determine the store layout, product presentation and services offered. We tailor our gift shop presentation to the needs of each hospital client.

Before we propose a gift shop layout, we evaluate the hospital's specialty, review its demographics and ethnic mix, and most importantly, we find out from the hospital what types of products and services they want represented in the gift shop. We successfully link with a number of clinical specialties, such as orthopedics or obstetrics, to provide support merchandise in the gift shop that doctors are recommending to their patients. Ultimately, the goal is to provide an enhanced customer service experience to the patient, offering one-stop shopping within the hospital — visit your doctor and leave with support merchandise that is prescribed, all within the same trip to the hospital.

Tony: The idea of healthcare-related products in the gift shop: Is that a relatively new trend? How does that fit with the history of what you've been doing?

Kim: It's definitely an emerging trend. In years past, our gift shops were really operating independently of the hospital, and we did not link with the clinical specialist. However, as administrators are becoming more concerned with patient satisfaction, we have responded by linking with the orthopedic clinics by offering specialized leg lifts, or obstetrics by offering breast pumps, or offering book titles that are published by the on-site doctors.

If an item or program is important to the hospital, it's important to us. If the hospital embraces the green initiative, we will offer a stronger selection of eco-friendly merchandise, such as dye-free bath and body lotions, soy candles and organic newborn blankets. Also, in response to the healthy living trend, we are offering a stronger selection of healthy snacks, trail mixes and sugar-free and fat-free products within our consumable department. These products, coupled with an increased assortment of juices, vitamin water and green tea, provides the consumer a health-conscious alternative.

Tony: What are the challenges of existing gift shops? There must be 4,000 to 5,000 of them, and many, if not the vast majority, are run by auxiliaries. What's the state of auxiliary-run shops, and why do you see administrators turning to you?

Kim: With hospital-run gift shops, administrators are finding it difficult to attract knowledgeable gift shop staff and volunteers. They often compromise by reducing the gift shop's operating hours or merchandise assortment, which decreases sales and customer satisfaction. Operating the gift shop can be an administrative burden to the hospital, requiring additional resources to either oversee the volunteers or payroll expense to staff the gift shop. And in volunteer-run gift shops, it is difficult for the volunteers to keep a full staff who can keep the gift shop open every day, including holidays and weekends.

Administrators are turning to us because we are retail experts in hospital gift shop management, allowing administrators to focus their attention on achieving excellence in patient care and not worry about the gift shop operation. The gift shop is the first impression to guests of a hospital and in today's competitive healthcare market, all avenues must be professionally managed to best reflect the image of the hospital. To have a gift shop with limited inventory, limited hours of operation or staffed with employees who are not customer-focused does not represent the hospital favorably.

With regards to volunteers, we embrace the tradition of volunteer-run gift shops by encouraging volunteers to continue working in the gift shop when we begin managing it. Volunteers choose their hours and the duties they perform, always backed by a paid Lori's staff member. In addition, all hospital volunteers and auxiliaries working in the gift shop or within the hospital receive a twenty-percent discount on eligible gift shop purchases. Other times, when the gift shop does transition from the volunteers to us, the volunteers are repositioned into other areas of the hospital that are in need of their support. Bottom line, we all want the volunteers to feel welcomed.

To further reinforce our commitment to the volunteer or auxiliary groups, we are more than willing to keep the same name of the gift shop that has been a tradition at the hospital for decades. We are proud to manage The Atrium gift shop at Yale-New Haven Hospital in Connecticut, the Rose Tree Gift Shop at Advocate Christ Medical Center in Illinois and The Rainbow Gift Shop at Abington Memorial Hospital in Pennsylvania.

Tony: What's coming in the next ten to fifteen years for the industry?

Kim: Hospitals will continue to develop retail marketplaces within their campuses, which will not only provide a strong revenue stream to the hospital, but having a cohesive retail model will ultimately benefit the visitors, patients and hospital employees by affording them the opportunity to purchase additional products and services at the hospital. You will see a greater linkage to the clinical staff by offering products that the doctors are recommending — and what better way to increase customer satisfaction than by providing the customer the opportunity to purchase a breast pump, for example, without ever leaving the hospital campus?

We continue to offer additional services in the gift shop such as selling stamps, local movie tickets, theme park tickets, massage therapy coupons and even hair salon coupons, if those services are offered on campus. We also offer a customer loyalty program in which all guests of the hospital accrue points and earn gift certificates to the gift shop.

Tony: In terms of getting a specific breast pump, for example, linking to the clinical staff, how do you achieve that in a hospital environment?

Kim: In the early stages of establishing a partnership with the hospital, we ask the administrators what they would like to see in the gift shop. Each gift shop is unique but backed by twenty-seven years of management experience. Our buying power allows us to offer an outstanding selection of preferred brands. So, if the hospital is recommending a specific brand of breast pump, a mineral-based lotion for cancer patients, or hospital logo apparel, because of our size, we can provide just about any item that is requested by administration.

Tony: What attributes are administrators focused on?

Kim: Administrators contact us for a variety of reasons when their gift shops are not meeting their expectations. A top request is extending the operating hours and the need to be open on weekends and holidays. Others are very concerned with the need to offer a stronger merchandise assortment and better inventory management. Others have been operating in the red and are looking forward to earning a profit in the gift shop by outsourcing.

Our goal is to provide a gift shop that is a true asset to the hospital while relieving the hospital of all management headaches. By assuming responsibility for all buying, staffing, merchandising and accounting functions, Lori's offers the ideal solution and frees up hospital resources to focus on patient care. In summation, hospitals are contacting us because they desire professionally run gift shop operations that embrace the values of their hospitals.

Tony: We've heard accolades about the Zen & Now Shop in Chicago. Is that the store that's carrying the eco-friendly product line?

Kim: Yes. We opened a new concept shop at Northwestern Memorial Hospital at the Prentice Women's Center in Chicago. Zen & Now embodies an eco-friendly design and offers complimenting health and wellness products. Everything in the gift shop supports the green initiative of the hospital, from the bamboo floors to a full assortment of organic clothing, mineral-based cosmetics and edible fresh fruit arrangements. We have created an oasis where mind, body and soul unite.

CHAPTER 9

THE HOSPITAL RESORT

When we hear the word "hospital," what is our first reaction? It's generally not a positive one. Hospitals are places where people go when they are sick or injured. Few people associate the word "hospital" with comfort or a sense of ease and well-being. And, at least part of that unease comes from *what* and *how* things happen at hospitals.

Patient comfort was not always a trivial concern. When Hippocrates founded the first hospital in Greece in approximately 400 BC, his philosophy was simple and profound: Surround patients with ample reasons to live and many will opt to do just that. Hippocrates did not have much science on his side with which to cure people, but his philosophy about care was correct. One's physical health has a great deal to do with one's state of mind.

The modern hospital model, conversely, has developed into an institution with a great deal of science on its side, though the amenities that give patients a reason to live are sometimes lost, and the patient as the principal purpose for the institution's existence is sometimes forgotten.

But that norm is quietly changing.

Again, we can thank the Baby Boomers, for whom personal care is a priority. It only makes sense that a generation willing to spend billions of dollars in the quest to look and feel better will expect its hospital experiences to be upgraded as well. If an elective procedure must be paid for out of pocket, why not stay in a hospital suite that resembles a four-star hotel? If comfort and personalized care is the norm, why shouldn't hospitals adapt to it?

Before Boomers came along, birth was accomplished with the mother isolated from her family and put in a drug-induced haze. Birthing has now become a more rewarding experience for all involved. And when the Boomers' parents aged, hospice care improved noticeably as well. Consumer-driven initiatives in healthcare are always effective out of economic necessity for the healthcare institutions.

Many hospitals are, in fact, already responding to that consumer directive. Bright colors, flat-screen TVs and artwork are brightening some of those drab hospital rooms. Room service and real restaurant-quality food are replacing boring cafeteria food. Internet service is becoming a standard feature. In short, proactive hospitals are recognizing that consumers with options care about amenities. And where are such things more important than in a hospital, where the emotional experience can be so overwhelmingly negative?

Nowhere is this change more evident than in the demise of the semi-private room. "Single rooms have become the industry norm," says Mike Romano of *Modern Healthcare* magazine. "Almost everything being built now is single rooms."[1]

The change to private rooms is not purely amenity-driven. The reality of modern medicine is that privacy laws and persistent pathogens like MRSA make sharing hospital rooms physically and legally challenging. The ability to perform many procedures on an outpatient basis has freed up space as well, leaving more rooms for single inhabitants. But the driving force behind the shift is that modern patients who are physically and emotionally vulnerable want privacy and comfort.

The patient as both provider and payor has changed the way hospitals look. Many world-renowned hospitals have even created luxury suites for consumers who are willing to pay more out of pocket for top-notch accommodations. Such facilities as Johns Hopkins in Baltimore, Cedars-Sinai in Los Angeles, Massachusetts General in Boston and Mount Sinai in New York City have created "pamper suites" that provide amenities similar to those found at upscale hotels.

Hospital food, which traditionally vied with airline food as the low standard for edibility by most people, has become an indispensable part of the more consumer-friendly hospital environment. Institutional food, traditionally prepared in mass quantities, has been replaced by food that's prepared to order. In addition, many hospitals have added vegetarian and low-fat options.

Food costs, naturally, have risen, but not nearly as much as you might expect. At Holy Spirit Hospital in Camp Hill, Pennsylvania, officials reported that food costs had in fact decreased because patients were throwing away less food. In the process, they noted that patient satisfaction had risen from thirty-eight to seventy-one percent.[2]

Most hospital patients aren't yet having their meals prepared by chefs, but certainly the image of generic, gray hospital food has been replaced by fare that's fresh and engaging, and appetizing to a more discerning consumer.

ASK THE EXPERT

George Naddaff is considered by many to be the guru of franchising in America. George began his career in food service in 1967, when he cofounded International Foods. In 1988 George founded New Boston Chicken, Inc. and served as its Chairman and CEO until 1993. George has been significantly involved with several other successful concepts including the founding of Mulberry Child Care Centers, Living and Learning Schools, Sylvan Learning Centers and VR Business Brokers, the nation's largest business brokerage franchise with over 350 offices. Today George is Chairman and CEO of UFood Restaurant Group, a "better for you," publicly held company that operates and franchises fast-casual restaurants featuring healthy meals.

Tony: How did you come up with the concept of healthy fast food?

George: It was first by accident, but in a sense we're all about taking from life's experience. I was driving through Watertown, Massachusetts, and saw this incredible, long line of people outside a fast food location. I couldn't wait to get in line and see what the excitement was about. To make a long story short, when I finally got into the restaurant, there was this huge menu with the nutritional values under each of the menu items. It was the first time I'd ever seen menu labeling. That was four or five years ago.

When I saw this concept I knew it was different and I began looking at the consumers in the line. It was a potpourri of humanity. I saw people in spandex, business people, some nurses from the local hospital. It was really quite unique. I spent the next hour observing people eating, and over the next several weeks I began to visit during lunch and dinner. I said to myself, "This has some serious legs."

Tony: You're looking at hospitals as potentially great locations for your restaurants. How would you rate the food they're offering?

George: I think hospitals lived in the Stone Age for quite some time in terms of nutrition. Today the movement is for wellness — what can we do for our patients and the people who visit our hospitals? I think hospitals have finally recognized that they have to do a lot more than just the things they've been doing.

Tony: Why is the health food movement important?

George: Three hundred sixty-five thousand people die each year from obesity, but there are more gyms in this country than anywhere else in the world. You have people asking for better foods. There are more people running up and down the streets of America. Why? People want to live longer, and this is a movement whose time has come. There's nothing as powerful as an idea whose time has come.

Tony: What's the difference between UFood Grill food and fast food?

George: We're serving the same kinds of food that people eat every day. For example, we have a bison burger with lean cheese. You can have your burger. You want fries? Our fries are not fried in fryers; we air fry them, so you can have your fries. We're giving consumers what they normally eat every day except these meals are prepared healthier, with healthier sauces and recipes. We spent four years perfecting, defining and refining this.

Tony: Is this just a fad? Where are consumers going to be in five or ten years?

George: Look at Whole Foods. They're creating this organic, natural product line. They're the groundbreakers. They say they put their locations where there are educated consumers. We follow them because they're the groundbreakers — educating Americans on how to eat better. That has a spillover effect, so when people are traveling or near their offices they're going to be searching for better foods, and we're going to be right there.

Technology has also been upgraded, in some facilities, beyond the introduction of bigger televisions. A leading supplier of patient room technology, GetWellNetwork, has introduced an interactive software program that allows patients to access, from their bedsides, a host of communication, educational and entertainment resources that are integrated into the care delivery. Patients can thus participate more directly in their own care or communicate with the outside world, e.g., accessing their health information, providing pain assessment and feedback, ordering meals, accessing the Internet, texting with hospital staff and visiting entertainment channels.

Internet access through systems like GetWellNetwork also provides opportunities to access the hospital's online store. "Giving access to the online store from the patient's bedside is a wonderful convenience for patients, allowing us to deliver a better hospital experience — one that is becoming increasingly expected by patients," says David Bennett,[3] director of Web resource services for the Medical University of South Carolina, which uses GetWellNetwork in conjunction with a Paquin Healthcare retail strategy.

Is medicine going in a direction that favors the wealthy? The practice of offering extra amenities for those willing to pay more is hardly discriminatory. These are facilities that have upgraded patient amenities in general, but acknowledge that there are patients willing to pay hundreds or even thousands of dollars extra for hospital rooms that more closely resemble four-star hotel suites.

The realization that hospitals are places to be avoided has led many institutions to rethink their involvement in the entire patient care continuum. In March 2006, Henry Ford Health System in Michigan announced that it had hired Gerard van Grinsven as president and CEO of one of its new hospitals. That van Grinsven was a qualified corporate leader was undeniable, but it was his twenty-four years in management for The Ritz-Carlton that caught the media's attention. And Henry Ford management acknowledged as much. "Our goal is to offer first-class service to match our world-class medical care," said Henry Ford Senior Vice President Robert Riney at the time.[4]

ASK THE EXPERT

A recognized expert on customer relations and satisfaction, Judy Foley is the CEO of Balance Concierge. With extensive healthcare and consulting experience, Judy started Balance Concierge after successfully serving in several leadership roles with one of the Midwest's most respected health systems. As Director of Patient and Guest Services for Sparrow Health System in Lansing, Michigan, she designed and implemented the health system's first concierge service for physicians, nurses, patients, staff and volunteers. The program has helped make Sparrow the employer of choice, surpassing General Motors as the largest job provider in mid-Michigan. In addition, Judy's expertise in customer relations resulted in dramatic increases in customer satisfaction and retention. Her Patients First initiative of service excellence continues to deliver exceptional patient and staff satisfaction today.

Tony: How did you get into this business, and what services do you provide?

Judy: I had the idea about six years ago and brought it into the healthcare facility where I was then working. What triggered my thinking about it was that we were implementing numerous strategies to improve patient satisfaction and attempting to get the employees involved in that effort. I'm seeing this stressed-out employee base — a mother, for example, who finally has a day off and at 5:30 a.m., she gets a call because a coworker has called in sick. People in healthcare are very dedicated; for many healthcare workers, it is a calling. So, they drop what they're doing and come in to work even though they have a full to-do list that day. I thought, why not offer some services to help alleviate this stress and help people balance their lives a little bit more?

Tony: What type of concierge services do you offer? Are they for employees only?

Judy: Actually, my services are offered to employees, patients, physicians, family members of patients and volunteers. But I believe it is best to start out by offering the services to your employees first. I recommend that highly because in healthcare we continue to ask employees to do more, and they need some relief to help them put more balance in their lives.

Services we offer fall into four categories: wellness, dependent care, recognition and typical convenience services like dining, entertainment, making reservations, picking up movie tickets at a discount and providing automotive services. People can drop their car keys off with the concierge and pick up their cars at the end of their shifts and the oil will have been changed, the tires will have been rotated, the windshield could have been repaired, and all while they were on the job. We want to be able to offer a service that allows people to come to work at the start of their shifts and hand their to-do lists to somebody else. This helps them stay focused at work and allows them time with their families in their off-time.

Tony: What's the most appreciated service?

Judy: Services that fall in the automotive category are very popular. The personal services like dry cleaning, too. A real big hit was the take-home meal, because these folks, particularly those in the clinic, work twelve-hour shifts. They can leave their shifts and take home three or four dinners to go.

Tony: What's the wildest idea you've ever run into?

Judy: This story isn't wild, it's touching. We had a girlfriend and boyfriend both in the hospital at the same time. One was dying of cancer and they wanted to have a wedding before she passed away. We helped arrange for that wedding and she passed away shortly after.

Tony: Who pays for this?

Judy: The hospital contracts with me for an established fee, then the employees, patients and families, physicians and volunteers are able to access the services of the concierge at no cost to them. The only cost is what pay for the service they request. For instance, if they choose to have their oil changed and their tires rotated, they'll pay that fee. However, all the services we offer have been arranged for with a discount.

Tony: What percentage of hospitals do you estimate offer concierge service, and what percentage should offer it?

Judy: The most recent statistic between 2005 and the present is that the percentage of hospitals offering these services grew from three percent to five percent. I project that in the next five years that number will grow upwards to ten percent or more.

Tony: I think it may grow even more rapidly based on the requirements we're placing on employees and the things we're asking them to do.

Judy: I couldn't agree more. You're looking at a competitive edge of being able to attract and retain talent and reduce stress levels. On the patient side, you're enhancing the patient experience, increasing loyalty, perhaps improving your fund development; with volunteers, strengthening those relationships; with the physicians, strengthening those loyal relationships as well. Looking at it from a human resources perspective, you're reducing turnover, seeing the expenses you save and seeing new levels of employee satisfaction.

CONCIERGE HEALTHCARE SERVICES

Some physicians have adapted to the reality of a consumer-driven healthcare industry as well, converting their practices in both size and features. With a limited number of patients, such doctors are offering twenty-four-hour phone access, same- or next-day appointments, comprehensive physicals, luxurious offices and personalized wellness plans. This trend, which has been adapted thus far by about 500 physicians nationwide, is known as "concierge" healthcare.

Such practices often require out-of-pocket retainers and effectively exclude patients of modest means, and the beneficial effect on patient health has yet to be proven. And with 300,000 primary-care doctors nationally, the impact on the healthcare industry has been minimal thus far. But this trend further illustrates that many consumers are willing to spend considerable expense not necessarily for better health, but for the amenities that come with personalized service.

CHAPTER 10

A HOSPITAL RETAIL PLAN

In this chapter an optimum retail plan will be presented for a fictional hospital based on real-world plans that have been developed and implemented by leading healthcare institutions in the United States by Paquin Healthcare Companies. While the actual numbers and specifics will vary from institution to institution, the principles, used to build a retail service line, remain the same.

Let's say you're an executive at a medical facility called Wellcare Hospital. You've worked in the industry for more than twenty years, and you recognize the trends in healthcare that make turning a profit increasingly difficult. You're familiar with the quote of noted consultant Peter Drucker, who said of hospitals: "Even small healthcare institutions are complex, barely manageable places. Large healthcare institutions may be the most complex organizations in human history."[1]

Immediately, you realize that the healthcare industry must change soon, and that your institution must change rapidly just to survive. Can you continue a mission-based operational plan, serving your community, without bankrupting your institution? Is there a way off the sinking ship that is the existing American health-care system?

This is where a consumer-focused, retail healthcare business plan becomes a key part of your strategy. The need to understand consumers and their expectations has never been greater.

It's not a one-size-fits-all solution, though many of the trends being addressed are common to the industry. This plan does not contain every detail required to implement a retail healthcare program; however it presents an overview of what's required for a successful retail plan.

We begin with simple math. A survey of your hospital employees finds that the majority support the idea of creating retail opportunities within the hospital. Another study shows that your employees, most of who are upwardly mobile professionals, each spend more than $15,000 every year on retail.

With more than 3,000 full- and part-time employees at Wellcare Hospital, there is the potential for millions in sales to a captive audience. Your employees already account for eighty percent of the sales in your volunteer-operated gift shop. With expanded product lines, a professional sales staff, marketing guidance and longer retail hours, your in-house business could take a healthy share of that existing market.

Last year, Wellcare Hospital recorded more than 150,000 patient encounters. Between these patients, their visitors and the hospital employees, we can project millions in high-margin retail revenue potential.

This added, high-margin revenue would help ensure that the rest of Wellcare Hospital, that vast and incalculably complex business organism, could continue to serve both its mission of community health maintenance *and* remain solvent.

Knowing your local market helps you properly market your products and services. The local area is your primary customer base, so if you provide for them what they need, they will remain loyal and reward your effort.

Once you've decided to move Wellcare Hospital into the retail healthcare field there are a number of necessary steps to organize your facility into an effective retail operation. Following are the essential steps needed to make a successful transition — one that benefits both the hospital and the community.

THE CLINICAL CONNECTION

It's not a question of whether patients are going to buy healthcare products; it's a question of where they will buy them. The first step in converting a traditional hospital into a retail healthcare operation is establishing the clinical connection, ensuring communication between the retail operation and your clinical staff. Caring for patients within the hospital has always been part of the facility's mission; with the clinical connection, you'll be ensuring their health away from Wellcare Hospital as well.

Medical professionals who recoil at the notion of being involved in retail healthcare are missing the greater benefit. By establishing a clinical connection and involving the hospital staff in the retail operation, patient outcomes are improved; this serves both the patients and the hospital, which can continue to function at a high level due to increased revenue.

Conducting education sessions hosted by the retail staff and attended by all medical professionals would both familiarize the staff with products and establish dialogue between clinical and retail staff members. With a steady dialogue, clinical staff could make recommendations and learn about new product lines. Rather than recommend products to patients and send them to unknown and questionable retail outlets, your team could assure that product solutions are provided to enhance patient outcomes.

Remember, a patient who is unaware that a product is available at the hospital store will purchase it elsewhere.

In traditional retail, the dressing room is the area where purchasing decisions are made. In the hospital environment, the clinical visit is the equivalent of the dressing room experience. Buying products directly from Wellcare Hospital that are recommended by staff ensures that the patient is getting the right product at a fair price, with the correct information on product usage and without having to make subsequent visits to other retailers.

For example, Mrs. A has been diagnosed with cancer by her doctor at Wellcare Hospital. She's currently undergoing chemotherapy and her oncologist recommends she purchase a non-metallic deodorant. There are three potential outcomes from this recommendation:

1. She may never purchase the deodorant and will instead continue to use a product that is not the best for her health.

2. She may drive to a traditional retail store to buy the product that's best for her.

3. She purchases the deodorant recommended by her clinician as she's leaving the hospital following her appointment.

Clearly, Mrs. A is best served when Wellcare Hospital has a retail healthcare component and a direct clinical connection.

To best implement the clinical connection, in addition to educational sessions for the staff, feedback sessions and new product introductions, Wellcare Hospital needs to institute the following practices:

- When a patient is discharged, nurses use a product form outlining products the patient should purchase at the hospital's store.

- Keep track of purchasing trends and an eye open for new product needs.

- Provide the same high-quality service to hospital employees that the general public receives. This is your initial client base — the people who will return as well as make recommendations. Send notes or emails thanking staff for utilizing the store.

- Develop a hospital mission statement that focuses on patient outcomes.

- Place product samples in the clinical locations — at a window display, a kiosk or the nurses' station.

- Build a database and develop a direct-marketing campaign to connect directly with patients.

- Develop e-commerce technology that allows patients to purchase products directly.

DETERMINING YOUR PRODUCT SELECTION

Healthcare facilities have three defined buying groups: patients, employees and visitors.

There are many factors to consider when operating a retail healthcare operation, but none is more important than the product line.
Products define the retail element just as services define the clinical aspect of the hospital, and the two are reflective of each other. So,
how does Wellcare Hospital determine which products it will need?

Product lines are a predictive science, not just guesswork. First,
there are core product categories that fit the predictive needs of the
three core buying groups. These are convenience items, healthcare
products, gifts and florals. Second, patient treatment trends and
traffic in certain facilities within the hospital help determine product placement.

In choosing products, the hospital should look for innovative brands
that are difficult to find in traditional retail outlets. Clinical staff can
contribute to this selection process. Staying abreast of new product
development is important; new products should constantly be integrated into the retail operation while maintaining the core products.

Products and merchandise can be found through a number of
sources including the *Hospital Buyer's Vendor Guide*, provided by
Paquin Healthcare Companies; suggestions from the clinical staff;
research into what other hospitals sell successfully; health and medical publications; trade shows; and the Internet.

Among the issues to address in determining Wellcare Hospital's
initial product line, as well as while maintaining and augmenting it,
are how well the products will sell, shipping costs and whether the
products will require technical support. Additional factors include
the margin of profitability, the shelf life of perishables, the stocking
of seasonal items, vendor qualifications and the potential liability
of products.

STAFFING AND THE DIRECTOR OF RETAIL

The first hire at your new retail enterprise will be the Director of Retail, whose job includes shaping the retail vision of the hospital, advancing the vision of the hospital's staff and volunteers and managing all aspects of its retail operations.

The retail operation's staffing should reflect the same commitment to patient service and community health as the hospital. Hiring should be based on retail experience, attitude, knowledge of healthcare or aptitude to learn, dependability, ambition, personality and willingness to buy into the retail mission.

Background checks and references are suggested, as are a dress code and a thirty-day training period. The structuring of the staff for a successful retail operation is important, and consultants like Paquin Healthcare can provide the hiring, training essentials and organizational guidelines for this endeavor.

E-COMMERCE

Selling products via the Internet is an essential element of retail healthcare, as it's become an essential element of almost every industry seeking to maintain its customer base. According to the most recent Shop.org study, online sales will exceed $200 billion this year. Other studies have shown that more than sixty-five percent of American adults continue to look for health-related information on the Internet.

Many people use the Internet to seek healthcare information, and an e-commerce site will allow such consumers to access information and products offered by Wellcare Hospital. The site can be both an advertisement and an extension of the hospital's retail selling plan.

Establishing an e-commerce site requires minimal capital investment, particularly compared to a traditional brick-and-mortar store.

The technology to create the site is readily available and affordable. The site itself must be professional, functional and easy to navigate, with pictures of each product. The site must also have a secure server for encrypting credit card information.

Product selection is important. Knowing that the Internet is an almost limitless marketplace, consumers want choices. This means carrying a wide variety of inventory that directly correlates to the store inventory.

Having an e-commerce site means that the virtual store will be open all the time. A toll-free telephone number and email contact must be established and must be staffed twenty four hours a day, seven days a week — meaning that customer service for the e-commerce site, while virtual, must actually be more prompt and reliable than at the hospital's store.

Because the e-commerce component of the business is complex, hospitals frequently outsource the operation. A third party that provides the technology, purchases the products, maintains inventory and provides customer service for a portion of the revenue will ensure a more efficient process and limit financial risk. Third-party providers are already serving other retail healthcare operations and thus have advanced systems to manage every aspect of the business.

In developing the e-commerce site, marketing must be considered. Potential consumers who are not patients will have no knowledge of your site unless several steps are taken.

These include:

- Setting up search engine registration using the hospital name and products the store carries.

- Using press releases to announce the store's opening.

- Creating a link from Wellcare Hospital's home page to the store site.

- Building email databases using sales or patient information so potential customers can be directly contacted.

- Handing out cards bearing the e-commerce site's address to patients, visitors and staff.

- Listing the e-commerce site on all advertisements, official releases and billboards.

- Integrating the e-commerce site with the existing Web site as often as possible.

- Informing exiting patients of the online as well as in-store availability of products.

- Posting new baby pictures on the Wellcare Hospital Web site; these pages could carry e-commerce reminders.

THE LOYALTY PROGRAM

Loyalty cards are an essential part of Wellness Hospital's retail healthcare program. There are a variety of loyalty cards and programs. Membership cards require consumers to pay fees in exchange for discounts and special promotions. Partnerships can be established with Visa or MasterCard, and a percentage of purchases can be provided to the hospital. There are also point-accrual customer loyalty programs.

The retail plan recommends a loyalty point accrual system for Wellcare Hospital. It's the most common system, and it's popular with consumers because there are no fees. Purchases simply accrue points for consumers, who can accumulate enough points to make further purchases at the hospital store or Web site. In addition, the data required to obtain a loyalty card can be used to directly market to customers — with the proper privacy protection provided, of course.

DIRECT MARKETING

Direct marketing will allow Wellcare Hospital to stay in contact with former patients, but moreover it will allow Wellcare to target specific audiences with specific products and services.

Direct marketing has a huge advantage over the brand-awareness campaigns traditionally embraced by hospitals. By reaching out to consumers and targeting them based on their needs or preferences, Wellcare Hospital will generate transactions without waiting for consumers to actually walk into the facility.

As part of direct marketing, patients can sign up for information on products and services directly related to their conditions and concerns. They can fill out checklists of information they would like to receive regarding products. Information can also be gathered from other avenues such as hospital services, membership groups, employee organizations and support groups.

Direct marketing will increase consumer visits to the store and Web site, as well as create interest in specific, targeted products.

MARKETING

Retail healthcare marketing is based on targeted, internal and external, direct communication with the appropriate audience.

There are fundamental concepts in retail healthcare marketing, and these can be applied to the specific needs of Wellcare Hospital and its target audience.

Wellcare already produces a newsletter, both in print and electronically, but the new newsletter will contain a link to the e-commerce site, and the retail staff will provide information about new products in addition to the existing articles written by hospital staff. The revised newsletter will also contain store hours and its toll-free telephone number.

Every opportunity should be taken to cross-promote the hospital and its retail operation. Patients should be made aware of both the store and the e-commerce site, and every store and e-commerce customer should be reminded of services offered at the hospital. Cross-promotion materials include flyers, catalogues and mailers. Everything produced throughout Wellcare Hospital's various enterprises should have a unified theme: the hospital name and logo, the physical and Web addresses, and a standard color scheme and font.

The most critical aspect of retail healthcare marketing is the continuous communication and involvement of the clinical staff. The staff's one-on-one, daily involvement with patients is the most efficient means of communicating Wellcare Hospital's message, more than any mass communication could ever achieve. It's also an avenue for feedback on and ideas about expanding products and services. The marketing message is communicated to the appropriate audience by a trusted clinician within the retail space. It is the essence of a trusting, captive audience.

Several programs should be used by Wellcare Hospital to further the marketing process:

Focus groups: These can be used to better determine what patients are looking for in terms of products and services.

Panels and advisory boards: These are select individuals who meet on a regular basis to make suggestions regarding the retail operation. Clinical staff, retail staff, hospital management and volunteers can all serve in this capacity.

Acquiring information: Gathering information with patients and consumers not only opens lines of communication but allows for marketing based on interests and medical needs.

Loyalty cards: Not only do loyalty cards offer consumers discounts, they open up marketing opportunities.

Showing where the money goes: Customers want to understand how their purchases are benefiting the hospital, so posters showing which stores have contributed money to Wellcare Hospital can be posted.

Special programs: Free flu shots and blood pressure screenings are among the ways in which Wellcare Hospital can serve the community while drawing people into the retail space. Off-site promotions at fairs and public events are also opportunities to offer free services while distributing information on the retail operation, as well as collecting information useful in direct marketing.

SALES MANAGEMENT

Solid sales management is the foundation of all retail success, and healthcare is no exception. Hiring, training, measuring sales goals and management all must be implemented with the goal of running an efficient and profitable business. Key components of sales include:

- Knowing the clients and stocking the products they want and need.

- Training the staff to know the products and how to interact with customers.

- Collecting customer information whenever possible for targeted marketing.

- Continuing training and education as new products are introduced and new staffers are hired.

- Measuring results on daily, weekly and monthly bases by sales associate and by store. The most successful store and salesperson should represent the standard that all others strive to reach. High achievers should be rewarded with bonuses and trophies.

- Posting sales numbers where staffers can see them.

- Developing strategies to address underperforming stores or associates.

- Maximizing every selling opportunity. The hardest part of retail is getting the customer in the store, so a customer on hand should be greeted warmly, offered assistance and informed of items of interest. Multiple sales are the key to maximizing every transaction.

- Holding regular sales meetings. Retail is constantly evolving, with new employees, procedures and products. Make the meetings upbeat, positive and educational. Use time together as an opportunity to exchange information, motivate the staff and recognize high achievers.

VISUAL MERCHANDISING

Visual merchandising is the art of creating aesthetically pleasing displays that entice customers to make purchases.

Retail displays are any grouping of products on a physical structure such as a shelf or freestanding fitment. An attractive display will draw customers; an ability to examine and touch the item will make it more appealing. Every display should have a theme: similar items on the same shelf, expensive items displayed prominently. Displays are used to promote merchandise but also serve to entice customers into the store. Displays can be created in the entryway, in windows and on shelves. Maintaining the display to maximize its appearance should be done regularly.

CUSTOMER SERVICE

Customers are often willing to pay more for better service, and have greater loyalty to establishments where they're treated well. In retail healthcare, customer satisfaction links not only to retail success but to the overall well-being of customers. Excellent customer service is delivered through excellent store policies and high-quality customer-employee interactions.

Store policies must include convenient hours; a liberal return and exchange policy; a belief that "the customer is always right"; privacy and respect when dealing with customer purchases, given the intimate nature of many retail healthcare items; ample products; refreshments; a child-friendly atmosphere, possibly including a play area; and ease in speaking with staff, including name tags and polite phone manners.

Employee requirements must include stringent hiring guidelines; empowerment to accommodate customers whenever possible; thorough and continuous training; regular staff meetings; customer interaction protocol, including how to greet people in person and on the phone; and proper dress and comportment. There must also be recognition for outstanding sales associates.

STORE DESIGN

The fundamentals of store design will determine whether the operation can ensure an acceptable return on investment (ROI). The accepted ROI is twenty-four months, with eighteen months being optimal.

Wellcare Hospital's existing store will need to be expanded, which will require professional design with input from an architectural firm. With the hospital's fiscal future impacted by the store's success, the store must operate at maximum efficiency.

The store must be organized so products are easily seen and accessible. The merchandise must be displayed in attractive ways, using wall treatments, proper lighting, signs and organization to maximize appeal. The store must have a floor plan that allows people to move easily through the store, and it must be lit comfortably, with the goal of making even those with diminished vision to shop.

The storefront signage must stand out, be easy to read and understand, and compel people to enter the store. The storefront must be an open space with a transition zone when customers first enter, allowing them to adjust to the lighting and layout.

The interior must be comfortable. The longer a customer spends in a store, the more likely he is to make a purchase. Studies have also shown that shoppers prefer not to share an aisle with someone if the space is too narrow. In a hospital store, the aisles should be wide enough to accommodate walkers and wheelchairs. The layout should encourage free and easy movement throughout.

Checkout should be located near but not blocking the entrance/ exit, and should never be at the rear of the store.

For the floors, hardwood is preferable to carpet because it's easier to maintain. On the walls, colors, mirrors and fabric are encouraged to give a more engaging appearance. To create ambiance, the use of soft music and aromas can enhance the shopping experience.

TECHNOLOGY

Technology offers solutions for managing sales and profits, and there are four technological components that will be necessary when managing your operation. In healthcare, the implementation of retail technology is critical in several areas: improving inventory control, assuring proper pricing, analysis of sales and transactions and the management of outbound sales and marketing campaigns. Retail technology can measure results in an instant, but healthcare technology must rely on the complex organism that is the hospital for some of its information, so the process may be slower than at a "normal" store.

A retail healthcare management system (RMS) manages inventory, purchasing and vendors, and generates management reports. It's critical to have the RMS on a real-time basis and integrated with the point of sales (POS) system, and it should be integrated with other systems within the hospital as well, including the e-commerce site.

This will enable it to track all purchases. The RMS can even be integrated with the hospital accounting system.

The POS system both records purchases and removes purchased products from inventory, and integrates with the RMS to maintain accurate transaction records. In addition, a customer relationship management (CRM) system creates a database of customer purchases, preferences and transaction locations. A loyalty program is the best tool in developing a CRM system; the data collected enables all future marketing and represents trends in purchasing and product use.

Traffic counters should be installed in the store as well as the main entrance to the hospital. Measuring pedestrian traffic allows for analysis and improvement of retail strategies.

THE MEDICAL DAY SPA

As noted earlier in the book, the medical spa industry is the fastest-growing segment of the spa industry, exceeding $11 billion annually and operating at twenty- to thirty-percent profit margins. The key to revenue production is creating rooms that can be booked on an hourly basis and combining medical and spa treatments. This multi-layering of spa services has proven to generate as much as $200,000 from one room.

Medical spas differ from day spas in that the former are operated under the direction of physicians. This allows medical spas to perform more complicated and costly procedures, and because these are generally not covered by insurance, medical spas are mostly cash businesses, with prices dictated by the market and not by insurance companies. Many patients view medical spa treatments

as less-invasive, less-expensive alternatives to invasive surgical procedures.

The following services are appropriate for Wellcare Hospital's
medical spa:

- Massages (relaxation, therapeutic, sports, maternity)

- Facials

- Manicures/pedicures

- Chemical peels

- Microdermabrasion

- Laser hair removal

- Botox

- Cellulite treatments

Wellcare Hospital's medical spas can service patients, visitors, staff
and people in the community. By creating a second facility off-site,
the business can generate even more business. Again, all spa services will carry the message of Wellcare Hospital's retail healthcare
operation, and the spa will serve as both a referral point and an
ambassador for the main hospital in the community.

DATA OVERVIEW

On what information do we base these recommendations? A thorough study of surveys of Wellcare Hospital personnel, statistics
from location-specific market reports, traffic counts, consumer
retail surveys, competitive market analysis, patient census and other
sources all contribute to these conclusions.

Five other important research reports relevant to Wellcare Hospital's market have been produced. These reports are:

Health and beauty market potential: This report identifies market demand for health and beauty products and services among both adults and households.

Medical expenditures: This report details the total dollar amount and average amount per household spent for medical care and health insurance items including physicians, prescription drugs, eyeglasses and contacts, hearing aids and health insurance.

Demographic and income profile: This report summarizes the 2000 census, current estimates and five-year forecasts of household data to reveal trends in demographics and income, including the consumer dollar potential available for various retail categories.

Market profile: This provides an overview of key demographic characteristics and consumer spending patterns in the immediate area.

Tapestry segmentation area profile: The sixty-five market segments of the Community Tapestry system classify neighborhoods in the U.S. based on their socioeconomic and demographic composition. This report compares the top five segments in Wellcare Hospital's area to their national counterparts.

A sample of the demographic groups predominant in the vicinity of Wellcare Hospital, as detailed in the Tapestry Segmentation Area Profile, is enterprising professionals. These are young, highly educated working professionals. Single or married, these city-dwellers prefer newer neighborhoods with townhouses and apartments and would rather rent than own. Median household income is $65,000.

Their lifestyle reflects their youth, mobility and consumer clout. They're dependent on computers, cell phones and PDAs and travel for both business and pleasure. They practice yoga, take aerobic classes and run to stay fit.

Many of the local enterprising professionals are employees at Wellcare. Knowing that this demographic represents a significant segment of the local populace is useful in determining which services and products to offer.

Thorough research into the medical spa business in the area has revealed information about existing facilities, including services and products offered. For example, Sunshine Med Spa, which is three miles from Wellcare Hospital, offers such services as facials, massages, microdermabrasions, ultrasound, peels and treatments, laser hair removal, laser vein treatments, laser skin rejuvenation, Botox, Restylane, DPT treatments with Levulan, tattoo removal and IPL. The facility uses the brand name products SkinMedica, SkinCeuticals, Physiodermie and PCA.

At Wellcare Hospital, foot traffic studies reveal in excess of 450,000 people entering the main facility each year. Because there is no existing automated point of sale system in the hospital gift shop it's impossible to compare the foot traffic to the sales data, but because there is a high number of visits it's reasonable to anticipate high sales volume in an improved retail establishment.

Our patient demographic study has broken down these visits by purpose. Those 450,000 visitors to the main facility include: 143,000 for outpatient surgery, 26,000 for oncology, 80,000 for imaging, 80,000 for endoscopy, 8,000 for urgent care, 25,000 for lab services and 40,000 for the adjacent health club.

Our extensive employee survey revealed that eighty percent would buy their uniforms and scrubs at work if they were available; seventy-eight percent use vitamins; ninety-four percent purchase health and beauty aids at the local pharmacy; sixty-five percent use a health club; fifty-two percent used a spa in the past six months; eighty percent would prefer a payroll deduction to pay for services and products at work; and ninety-seven percent have home computers, most used for purchasing products online.

Remember, the staff is your first and most loyal customer base. The staff at Wellcare Hospital is a demographic that would seek the products and services being considered for the retail healthcare operation.

The clinical retail survey compiled a list of the products provided at no charge to patients at Wellcare Hospital. Staffers were also asked for suggestions of products they'd want to see available at the retail operation. The most common responses to the latter question included such staples as aspirin, vitamins and Tylenol as well as home traction units, electrical stimulation units and breastfeeding equipment.

PROJECT OVERVIEW

A scientific approach to assessing opportunity and designing a business plan was undertaken for the implementation of a retail plan. Using the information gathered regarding Wellcare Hospital and its community, we can compare those results with the aggregate data from previous projects to develop a realistic business plan.

Our objectives are to provide new, profitable revenue opportunities; improve patient satisfaction and wellness by extending the continuum of patient care; and offer a competitive advantage.

Based on those findings we can make following recommendations:

OPERATIONAL

The retail plan recommends the creation of a retail services depart-ment to consolidate all retail activities and revenue reporting. This department should be staffed by a paid retail workforce under the direction of a Director of Retail Services. This individual should have extensive retail experience and an entrepreneurial approach to implementing new ideas, and must be able to work closely with staff to ensure that the mission is understood and best practices are being implemented throughout the operation.

The retail component should operate under the same mission, vision and culture as the healthcare component. The Director of Retail Services will be responsible for coordinating retail through-out the existing systems within Wellcare Hospital, and the existing services within the hospital must embrace retail as a an additional service line with the same goal of extending the continuum of care and improving patient outcomes.

PRIVATE LABEL PRODUCTS

The retail plan recommends the deployment of exclusive, private-label products in all retail locations. Wellcare Hospital products will be different from conventional retail brands and will facilitate loy-alty to the hospital. Specific products should include vitamins, nutraceuticals, mineral cosmetics and natural skin care products. Products should be sourced from a reputable manufacturer.

These products should be deployed at all Wellcare Hospital facilities including fitness centers, physician offices, ambulatory centers, e-commerce sites, medical spas and any other appropriate retail outlets.

CUSTOMER LOYALTY

A comprehensive CRM strategy can be achieved through a loyalty card program while offering customers of Wellcare Hospital extended benefits and rewards for purchasing products and services. Points can be accrued for purchases. Patients will provide specific personal information to obtain their loyalty cards, which can be done at any Wellcare Hospital location. The CRM database will then allow Wellcare to market all retail initiatives including home care, medical spas, retail stores and e-commerce sites, as well as new services.

VIRTUAL AND DIRECT MARKETING

Virtual and catalogue opportunities will enable the retail operation at Wellcare Hospital to reach consumers wherever they are. Condition-specific online stores should be deployed; common conditions should include diabetes, rehab, home health, cardiology, personal care, employee uniforms and mom/baby.

E-commerce can be used as a tool for medical staff to connect patients with recommended products simply by registering online and customizing lists. Patients can then refer to their lists and shop from home, extending the health continuum beyond the hospital or clinic visits.

Staff should be trained to introduce the e-commerce concept to patients. Computers should be provided in the hospital, in both common areas and the store, to teach patients how to use the sites as well as provide access to those who don't own a computer.

Wellcare Hospital should partner with a firm to provide technology, order fulfillment and inventory management to reduce the initial capital investment. An outsourced direct-marketing program will provide a commission based on sales.

To further enhance customer convenience and remote accessibility, the retail plan recommends the deployment of a direct-marketing strategy for nutritional supplements. These programs can generate millions in revenue and can be placed on auto-replenish status, allowing for predictable and consistent results.

The direct-marketing initiative should be created to invite customers and patients to request information regarding health-specific products and nutritional supplements. Information can be gathered during the registration and check-in process as well as through participating clinics.

BRICK-AND-MORTAR LOCATIONS

Wellcare Hospital should assume ownership of its adjacent fitness centers, which are currently run by a health club operator. These centers can provide an anchor for many of the retail initiatives.

Once this is accomplished Wellcare should re-merchandise the retail areas within the fitness centers. Each center has an established member base, one that's identified as having a strong interest in health. In addition to the existing product lines, which consist mostly of apparel, the retail plan calls for the stocking of wellness products, as well as convenience and consumable items such as vitamins, protein shakes and powders, and nutritional bars.

Wellcare Hospital has a number of facilities where retail can be addressed. Let's take one of its wellness centers as typical, and then address the hospital's main facility, medical spa and cancer pavilion.

Wellness center number one has a constituency that's seeking a wider range of products that support healthier lifestyles, such as cookbooks and small fitness equipment. Relocating the member desk to the lobby will free space in the retail operation. A broader selection of existing products, a coffee area and the introduction of fitness nutrition items will ensure repeat sales.

The Wellcare Hospital gift shop should be redeployed as a marketplace store. As such it should contain trendy and innovative gifts as well as lifestyle and convenience items. The store should have the look and feel of a traditional retail operation with warm colors, consistent fixtures and engaging displays.

The strategic plan calls for at least 2,000 square feet for the establishment of a medical spa. An elegant and welcoming lobby sets the tone for the experience. Treatment rooms and relaxation spaces should be designed to maximize the sensory refreshment one should expect. Services would include massages, acupuncture/acupressure, facials, reflexology and manicures/pedicures, as well as microdermabrasion, injectibles and light therapy.

At the Wellcare Hospital cancer pavilion, a merchandising strategy should include "A Place for Her," which would include boutique items as well as items that will appeal to the health and image-conscious cancer patient. Specific items would include vitamins and nutraceuticals relevant to women's health, mineral cosmetics and natural skin care products for those undergoing cancer treatments, and an expanded line of gift, spa, jewelry and inspirational merchandise.

FINANCIAL SUMMARY

In its second full year of operation, the retail division of Wellcare Hospital should generate more than $14 million in gross sales. This assumes, of course, the creation of healthcare marketplaces and medical spas, as well as the implementation of the recommendations contained in this plan.

The net operating margin for the retail operation should be ten to twelve percent, with a higher amount realized in coming years. This estimate does not account for depreciation, interest or taxes.

The vast majority of revenues are directly related to patient care, and thus should be business-related income and have the option of operating under a not-for-profit structure.

An outsourced partnership arrangement is recommended for the e-commerce portion of the business. We project a ten-percent income for Wellcare Hospital from e-commerce revenues.

Partnering is also recommended for the vitamin direct-marketing program. This partner should take all financial risk, provide investment capital and guarantee pharmaceutical-grade vitamin products. We project a ten-percent income for Wellcare Hospital on direct-marketing revenues.

A detailed strategic plan should include listings of recommended products; projected expenses; projected earnings by facility; a financial summary for the wellness spas; a five-year financial outlook for all retail operations, capital requirements, operating plans, and staffing requirements; and space allocations for the implantation/expansion of recommended facilities.

The two-year net income for Wellcare Hospital should exceed $2 million; long-term net income should exceed $2.5 million annually.

ASK THE EXPERT

Charles M. Trunz III founded and was appointed President of Vivo Health, Inc. in 2007. Vivo Health, a subsidiary of North Shore-LIJ Health System, is focused on creating new services and businesses that enhance healthcare delivery throughout the New York metropolitan area. The company has embarked upon building businesses that include Vivo Health, a consumer health and wellness company, and the commercialization of resident intellectual capital. Charles was promoted in 2004 to the position of Regional Chief Operating Officer of North Shore-LIJ with responsibilities for the management of two tertiary hospitals, a children's hospital, behavior health services and outpatient ambulatory services. Prior to joining North Shore-LIJ, Charles led JPMorgan's investment banking operations as COO and CFO, among other senior leadership positions, over twenty-one years at the firm.

North Shore-LIJ is now one of the ten largest healthcare systems in the United States, serving an area with 5.5 million people.

Tony: Why is a retail strategy or even a consumer strategy something that's important to the North Shore-LIJ Health System?

Charles: First and foremost, our retail health strategy is meant to better support and service the patients of the North Shore-LIJ Health System across all of our fifteen hospitals, seventeen affiliated nursing facilities, and numerous ambulatory centers. We must extend the care continuum for our community, building relationships with our patients prior to acute events and after they are discharged — a word, by the way, that can be wrongly interpreted. We want to discharge patients from our facilities but never from our care.

Critical to this mission is providing wellness and preventative services that empower the patient, the consumer, the community to maintain their health. Our mission is to provide the highest quality "sick-care" for acute events and injuries, but it also is to keep our patients out of the hospital through "life-care."

Tony: Patient satisfaction and outcomes and experiences and financial considerations… How do you prioritize them?

Charles: The first priority is service. It's not about financial profit; it's about providing services that meet community and patient needs. Financial benefits will accrue only after we service our consumers and patients with compelling services and products, and with insightful information so they can make informed decisions about what product or service is right for them.

Tony: What kind of retail programs has North Shore-LIJ utilized, and if you could, what kind of retail would you use in the future?

Charles: Retail, until now, has not been a definitive strategy for the health system. I've been asked by Michael Dowling, our CEO, to analyze the health system's tangible and intangible assets and to develop new patient services that leverage these assets. Our access to consumers and patients, our clinical expertise, brand, market share, and our reputation are just some of the health system's assets. What we have found is that retail healthcare services deserve strategic focus similar to our clinical services. Working with Paquin and other best-in-breed, visionary partners, we are building retail services within a multi-year strategic framework.

Tony: How are you organized in terms of those retail enterprises? Are they integrated into each hospital or are they overseen by a separate organization?

Charles: Right now they're separate. However, we are now working to consolidate these functions under North Shore-LIJ Health System's new consumer health and wellness company, Vivo Health. We believe consistency, discipline and a dedication to understanding our consumer's wants and needs will build more meaningful operations for our community and a powerful brand centered on wellness.

Tony: What do you see as the challenges of changing the culture to one that's perhaps more proactive, similar to something you would find in the retail world?

Charles: The number-one priority is service. We cannot compromise the delivery or quality of products and services to our patients. And we need continual patient feedback, with the ability to alter products and services rapidly to meet their needs.

Tony: Will retail act in some ways as sort of an outreach service with locations not necessarily adjacent to existing hospitals?

Charles: Yes. The Vivo Health brand and business operations will service our patients and consumers on-site, locally and regionally. This will be accomplished by converting gift shops into Vivo Health marketplaces and establishing targeted retail pharmacies, specialty stores and services. And, of course, the operation will be anchored online with VivoHealth.com to address patient product, service and medical information needs.

Tony: What are the important factors with Internet services?

Charles: All aspects of healthcare have moved to a patient-centric model. The Internet is one significant driver of this industry shift away from a provider- and employer-centric model. As in other industries, the Internet, if not now, is quickly becoming the first place consumers research medical healthcare information, purchase their medical and health-related needs, and manage their overall health and wellness.

Couple this trend with electronic medical records and personal health records. Imagine the power of the Internet in the future, when a person's health information is globally accessible, integrated and shareable between health providers, caregivers and patients. The Internet will be the source by which the patient communicates with physicians, hospitals and, importantly, each other. In the meantime, it is now the number-one resource for making educated decisions about what services and products are needed to maintain their health. And Vivo Health is, on behalf of the community and the health system, working to ensure that we share our clinical insights and expertise.

Tony: A review of your Web site properties shows that North Shore is already seeing 300,000 visits per month.

Charles: Yes, and the system is working diligently to further enhance and build on our Internet presence. We are working with physicians, administrators and other clinicians to ensure that we have pertinent, timely and compelling content on our site that reflects the clinical quality of our health system.

Moreover, we see tremendous synergies between NSLIJ.org, VivoHealth.com and our intranet for better service, communication and education.

Tony: As you communicate some of these ideas to leaders within North Shore, what kind of response do you get?

Charles: In an organization of 38,000, as you can imagine, there are many voices. Initially responses were varied and the reception was a bit tepid. But I would also note that it took us at Vivo Health, Inc. time to find the right way to communicate our thinking. Once we stopped tripping over the message and understood and accounted for many important concerns, we found a very warm reception.

We are blessed to have a staff that is passionate about patient care. As soon as we connected the dots and demonstrated the patient and public-health benefits we found ourselves with overwhelming support. Moreover, working together, we identified old desires that weren't successful in the old models. In our new model, things such as on-site employee pharmacies, cardiac rehab and wellness services can be integrated into a sustainable model through Enterprises, Vivo Health and our new wellness center.

Tony: Charles, you've had an exceptional career in that you've worked in both healthcare and investment banking. How would you relate your investment banking experiences to what you're faced with now?

Charles: In both businesses the value proposition is the same: the patients and clients come first. We must provide products and services that are appropriate for our patients. At JPMorgan, we declined businesses if it was not in the best interest of the client. So in building any business, the foremost priority is understanding what the patient needs and determining the most effective way to serve that need.

Tony: If you were talking to another executive in a similar position at another hospital, what advice would you offer as they embark on a retail initiative?

Charles: First, a retail initiative needs a dedicated team. Not a big team, but one that is focused and that can interact with the larger organization. Second, one needs to candidly assess the strengths and weaknesses of their organization and any historical efforts to advance a similar agenda. Third, determine the critical success factors needed to ensure success. And understand that communication, almost above all else, is key. There should be a consistent message of priorities, services, time frames to deliver those services and expenses/capital required to execute. And, finally, one must also recognize that many hospitals do not have the experts necessary to execute and manage these retail initiatives. This is the reason we have a philosophy of partnership. As you know, we rely heavily on thought leaders and the experience of teams such as Paquin Healthcare to define, develop and execute the strategies I have discussed in this interview.

CONCLUSION

Healthcare is a national problem, with many Americans uninsured and many more underinsured. A system that treats illnesses provides wellness care, and one that can turn a profit, thus staying in business and continuing to serve the community, is a benefit to everyone. Just as consumers have adapted to the wealth of information available about maintaining their health, so too must the healthcare industry adapt to both these newly empowered consumers and the economic realities of this new healthcare economy.

Following the lead of its informed patients/consumers, the healthcare industry is slowly but surely shifting its focus from a reactive business that primarily treats patients to one focused on keeping people healthy. A preventative, retail approach will ultimately alleviate much suffering as well as reduce healthcare costs. Wellness is already a huge business, largely unregulated and unmodified by physician referrals and hospital branding. Medical facilities that adopt the retail healthcare plan provide better care for their patients while ensuring their own viability.

It isn't a matter of whether the established payment system will collapse or not; it's a matter of when it will happen. Short of a revolution in the current reimbursement-based healthcare industry, hospitals will continue to be economically unmanageable, even unexplainable, in their complexity. Retail, consumer-driven health-care ultimately offers the surest solution to this industry-wide economic crisis.

Hospitals are closing at an alarming rate, not for lack of patients but for lack of profitability. In becoming more profitable, financially viable hospitals serve communities as they serve themselves, remaining operational and providing care in an increasingly difficult environment.

Treating patients as customers, as informed and proactive consumers capable of making choices to benefit themselves, is ultimately a better system than the old one. The mission of all healthcare providers is to keep patients well; embracing the consumer movement is the best way to reach that goal while also ensuring the economic viability of the healthcare industry.

Adapting retail healthcare models outlined in this book, designed to the specifics of each medical entity, meets the needs of all interested parties: The community is served medically; retail healthcare products are vetted by medical professionals, ensuring safety and quality; and the hospital becomes an economically vital organization, allowing it to better serve its constituency.

Pushed by an aging Baby Boomer generation, and enabled by a wired Internet generation, consumers are flocking to healthcare products and services like never before in our history. Throughout the twentieth century, Americans created massive retail markets in homes, automobiles, clothing, electronics and more. As they now turn to their own health, consumers worldwide will create the largest retail movement in history.

Professional healthcare providers like major healthcare and hospital systems are the best qualified, and most deserving, to serve the needs of these consumers. A better-served consumer and a financially-stronger healthcare system is the ultimate win-win.

ENDNOTES

CHAPTER 3

1   Hammergren, John and Harkins, Phil, *Skin in the Game: How Putting Yourself First Today Will Revolutionize Health Care Tomorrow* (Wiley, 2008).

CHAPTER 4

1   Anderson, Chris, "The Long Tail," Wired, Oct. 2004, Anderson, Chris, *The Long Tail: Why the Future of Business Is Selling Less of More* (New York: Hyperion, 2006).

CHAPTER 5

1   Pew Research Center online poll, www.pewresearch.org, August 2000.

2   Costello, Daniel, "Hospital Has Aches, Pains Going Digital," *Los Angeles Times*, February 15, 2007.

3   Google BlogSpot, May 27, 2007.

4   Lohr, Steve, "Warning on Storage of Health Records," *The New York Times*, April 17, 2008.

5   Kanellos, Michael, "Health care's the ticket, Craig Barrett says," CNET News, http://news.cnet.com, April 13, 2005.

6   www.thehealthcareblog.com, September 16, 2007.

CHAPTER 9

1   www.bankrate.com, September 27, 2004

2   Mamula, Kris B., "Pittsburgh-area hospital food gets tasty, convenient upgrades," *Pittsburgh Business Times*, May 2, 2008.

3   www.getwellnetwork.com, February 20, 2008.

4   Gosselin, Gary, www.blog.mlive.com, January 31, 2008.

CHAPTER 10

1   Beatty, Jack, *The World According to Peter Drucker* (New York: Free Press, 1998).